Eat Green(ish)
Bananas to Lower
Blood Sugar

Brush Your Teeth
for Extra Immune
Support

Take Your Workout
Outside for Some
Vitamin D

Snack On Papaya
to Combat Low
Digestive Enzymes

GUT
HEALTH
HACKS

Avoid Artificial
Sweeteners That Might
Cause Gut Imbalance

Relax Your Mind
to Avoid Stomach
Issues

Practice Light
Yoga to Improve
Digestion

Eat Fermented
Foods for Healthy
Probiotics

200 WAYS GUT MICROBIOME AND TH!

LINDSAY BOYERS, CHNC Technical Review by **MURDOC KHALEGHI, MD**

Adams Media
New York   London   Toronto   Sydney   New Delhi

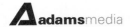

Adams Media
An Imprint of Simon & Schuster, Inc.
100 Technology Center Drive
Stoughton, Massachusetts 02072

First Adams Media trade paperback
edition July 2021

ADAMS MEDIA and colophon are
trademarks of Simon & Schuster.

For information about special discounts
for bulk purchases, please contact
Simon & Schuster Special Sales
at 1-866-506-1949 or business@
simonandschuster.com.

The Simon & Schuster Speakers Bureau
can bring authors to your live event. For
more information or to book an event
contact the Simon & Schuster Speakers
Bureau at 1-866-248-3049 or visit our
website at www.simonspeakers.com.

Interior design by Colleen Cunningham
Interior images © Getty Images

Manufactured in the United States of
America

1 2021

Library of Congress Cataloging-in-
Publication Data
Names: Boyers, Lindsay, author.
Title: Gut health hacks / Lindsay
Boyers, CHNC, technical review by
Murdoc Khaleghi, MD.
Description: First Adams Media trade
paperback edition. | Stoughton, MA:
Adams Media, 2021. | Series: Hacks |
Includes index.
Identifiers: LCCN 2021007343 |
ISBN 9781507216453 (pb) | ISBN
9781507216460 (ebook)
Subjects: LCSH: Gastrointestinal
system--Diseases--Diet therapy. |
Nutrition. | Self-care, Health--Popular
works.
Classification: LCC RC806 .B693 2021 |
DDC 616.3/30654--dc23
LC record available at
https://lccn.loc.gov/2021007343

ISBN 978-1-5072-1645-3
ISBN 978-1-5072-1646-0 (ebook)

CONTENTS

Chapter 4
PRIORITIZE YOUR MENTAL HEALTH 135

Chapter 5
MAKE SOME LIFESTYLE AND ENVIRONMENTAL CHANGES ... 177

INTRODUCTION

It's time to harness the amazing power of your gut! The health of your gut is vital to proper digestion, but that's only the tip of the iceberg. Your gut health is also tied to your immune function, your mental health, and your overall state of health and well-being. If your gut is out of whack, it's impossible to live your best life. But with so much information out there, it can feel overwhelming to try to sort through it all. Enter *Gut Health Hacks*.

In this book, you'll find two hundred hacks that help streamline everything there is to know about improving your gut health. You'll learn how to test your current gut function, the best dietary and lifestyle changes you can make to support your gut, and how you can improve your gut health by prioritizing your mental health.

The hacks in this book can not only lead to profound positive changes in your gut health, but they're also simple to incorporate. You can start by doing a handful of things at a time and working your way up to living a lifestyle that fully supports your gut health, or you can dive right in and give your life a complete gut health overhaul—the choice is yours.

Whether you're hearing about the importance of gut health for the first time or you're looking for some actionable steps to build on what you know, this book is here to keep your gut in tip-top shape.

Chapter 1

DO THE RIGHT TESTS TO ASSESS YOUR GUT HEALTH

If you've picked up this book, there's a good chance you already suspect that you're dealing with some gut issues. You might have digestive symptoms, like gas, bloating, diarrhea, and/or stomach pain, or some less obvious signs, like fatigue, headaches, rashes, and joint pain. More than likely you have a combination of both. But no matter what your personal gut concerns, the tests in this chapter will help you pinpoint what's going on and which factors are contributing to your issues.

You'll learn how to analyze your poop (don't worry, you don't have to touch it!), your skin, your digestive symptoms, and your body odor to uncover what's going on underneath the surface. You'll also learn how certain vitamins, minerals, and other nutritional compounds play a role in gut health and how to see if your body is getting adequate amounts of each. Some tests you can easily do at home, using common pantry ingredients like baking soda. Others require you to get your healthcare provider involved. You can start with one or do them all—the choice is yours. But once you uncover the things that may be contributing to your gut issues, you'll be ready to move on to the rest of the hacks in this book to restore your gut health.

#1

WATCH FOR SIGNS

This may not be a true "test," but taking note of your symptoms and identifying any patterns are vital parts of assessing your gut health. When you think of your gut, some symptoms point to a problem, like:

- Gas
- Bloating
- Constipation
- Diarrhea
- Stomach pain
- Heartburn
- Burping

But there are a lot of not so obvious signs too. If your gut is out of whack, it can affect your whole body in a negative way, leading to systemic symptoms that you might not even connect to your gut unless you're really paying attention. Some of these symptoms include:

- Cravings, especially for sugar or processed carbohydrates
- Unexplained weight loss or weight gain
- Anxiety
- Low mood
- Insomnia (difficulty falling or staying asleep)
- Skin rashes, acne, eczema, and/or psoriasis
- Poor concentration
- Chronic fatigue
- Any autoimmune disease

Keep in mind that these lists aren't all-inclusive. If you have any chronic, lingering symptoms that won't go away, keep track of them and see if you can find any correlations with your stress levels, diet, or overall lifestyle. If you can, fixing your gut may help solve, or at least improve, the problem.

JOURNAL IT!

A helpful way to connect any symptoms with your diet is to keep a food journal. Food journals help you identify which types of foods might be causing any persistent symptoms. It's really simple. All you have to do is write down:

- What you ate
- When you ate
- Any symptoms that you notice that day
- What your mood is like
- How much energy you have
- How well (or not well) you slept

It is important to write down everything you eat, no matter how small or insignificant you think it is. If you're sensitive to gluten, even a bite or two can cause symptoms, so you want to make sure you're accurately keeping track.

It's also important to write down every symptom or anything that feels "off." You may not connect certain symptoms with your digestion, but they may be closely related. For example, joint pain, poor memory, and fatigue are all signs of poor gut health, but they're not as obvious as other signs, like bloating or diarrhea.

Keep in mind that although many people have learned to live with nagging or uncomfortable symptoms, they're not normal. Even if you've been dealing with something for several years and you've learned to adapt, write it down. You may be able to connect it to something you're eating.

Another thing to keep in mind is that symptoms don't always show up right away. You may react to something you've eaten two or three days later, so pay attention to those connections and patterns too.

#3

ELIMINATE SOME FOODS

An elimination diet isn't a scientific test, but it's one of the most effective ways to identify food sensitivities. To follow a basic elimination diet, avoid the most common food allergens and gut irritants for a set period of time, usually thirty days. These allergens include:

- Gluten
- Soy
- Dairy
- Eggs
- Sugar and all sweeteners
- Grains (including corn and oats)
- Nightshade vegetables (white potatoes, eggplant, peppers, and tomatoes)
- Alcohol
- Caffeine (does not include herbal teas)

After the initial thirty days, which is called the removal period, move to the reintroduction phase. During this period, slowly bring the eliminated foods back into your diet, one at a time. For example, eat dairy for two to three days and then take note of any symptoms that return or flare up.

If you don't experience any symptoms, you can generally assume that your gut is tolerating that specific food pretty well and you can move on to reintroducing the next food. However, if you do experience symptoms, go back to your elimination diet for the next few days before reintroducing the next food.

The goal with an elimination diet is to identify which foods are a trigger for you and then to remove them from your diet, at least temporarily.

#4

LOOK BEFORE YOU FLUSH

After you've gone number two, you may just want to flush it and forget it, but looking at your poop can give you insights into the current state of your gut. An easy way to determine if your stool (and gut) is healthy is the Bristol Stool Chart. This chart breaks poop into seven types.

- Type 1 looks like separate hard lumps or pebbles. This type of poop indicates low levels of good bacteria or constipation.
- Type 2 looks like hard pebbles connected together, resembling a lumpy sausage. This type of poop signals constipation or can be a sign of irritable bowel syndrome.
- Type 3 looks like one solid poop, but with cracks on the surface. This indicates that you may be dehydrated, and constipation is likely, although it's still considered fairly normal.
- Type 4 looks like one smooth continuous log. This is an ideal-looking poop.
- Type 5 looks like individual blobs, but there are still edges on each piece. This is the start of diarrhea and shows that you may not be digesting food properly, especially if undigested food particles are present.
- Type 6 looks mushy with some lumps still present. This is a sign of increased transit time (the time it takes food to travel through the digestive tract) and can indicate a gut disorder.
- Type 7 is watery with no solid pieces at all. This can come from gut infections, either chronic or short term (like food poisoning), or eating something that doesn't agree with you.

While certain poop characteristics are considered normal, everyone is unique. Looking at your poop can help you figure out what's normal for you and when something seems off.

#5

CHECK FOR FLOATERS

Healthy poop sinks to the bottom of the toilet bowl quickly and quietly, without plopping or splashing. If your poop floats and/or contains pieces of undigested food that are floating around it, these are signs that something may be off with your gut.

Floating stool is most often a sign of malabsorption. Usually it means that you're not digesting fat properly, which can interfere with the proper absorption of all types of nutrients and leave you at risk of developing vitamin and mineral deficiencies.

But what causes malabsorption? Some common causes of floating stool are:

- Lactose intolerance
- Liver problems
- Intestinal disorders, like Crohn's disease

Your poop may also float if there's a lot of gas in your digestive tract. The gas gets trapped in the stool, making it more buoyant. Gas can come from innocuous things like eating a lot of high-fiber foods or eating too much in general, but it can also come from more serious things that need attention, like food intolerances or gut infections (*E. coli* or salmonella, for example).

Before you flush, take a look and check for floating poop. If you've recently started eating more fiber, that may explain the newly buoyant stool. In this case, it should settle as your body adjusts. However, if you've made no dietary changes and you're seeing floaters regularly, you may need to determine if you have any food intolerance or infection.

TAKE A WHIFF

Poop smells bad—there's just no way around it. A lot of things make your poop smell the way that it does, but it mostly comes down to the bacteria in it. Each of the different types of bacteria in your digestive system produces different gases. All of those gases are pretty unpleasant, but sometimes the smell is rancid. This happens to everyone once in a while, but if your poop is consistently clearing the room, there's likely a bigger issue at play.

Really smelly poop is often a sign of malabsorption—an inability to properly absorb nutrients from the food you're eating—which happens when your gut isn't functioning as it should. This can happen if you're eating something your gut doesn't like or if you have an underlying disorder like celiac disease, Crohn's disease, or an inflammatory bowel disorder.

Foul-smelling stool can also stem from a gut infection, whether it's viral, bacterial, or parasitic. When you have an infection, your gut becomes inflamed and you're more likely to experience smelly diarrhea along with cramps, bloating, and vomiting.

You should never expect your poop to smell *good*, but take a couple of whiffs before you flush. Pay attention to any major changes, and if the smell is getting rancid, your gut needs some extra care.

CARE ABOUT COLOR

Medium brown is the standard poop shade, but all shades of brown and even some green colors can be normal. The color of your poop changes with what you're eating—for example, beets will turn it reddish, while lots of leafy green vegetables will make it green—so you shouldn't be too concerned if what you see in the toilet doesn't always look the same.

Here is the meaning of different poop colors:

- Light green = Food is moving through your digestive system too quickly and bile doesn't have time to break it down. It could also mean you're eating a lot of green, leafy vegetables.
- White or light-colored = There's not enough bile in your stool. It could mean you have problems with your liver or gallbladder or a bile duct obstruction.
- Yellow (and possibly greasy) = You have excess fat in your stool, which could indicate you have a malabsorption disorder like celiac disease.
- Mucus-covered = You may have an overgrowth of bacteria in your digestive tract or an inflammatory condition such as Crohn's disease or colitis.
- Bright red = You have bleeding in the lower digestive tract, usually from hemorrhoids or an anal fissure.
- Deep red, black, or tarry = You have bleeding in the upper digestive tract. If you haven't eaten beets recently, which could account for the color, it's a good idea to check in with your doctor.

#8

SET YOUR TIMER

Did you know that, on average, it takes mammals about twelve seconds to poop? In a 2017 study in *Soft Matter* (yes, there is a scientific study on poop duration in a journal titled *Soft Matter*), researchers timed thirty-four different mammals, from cats to elephants, relieving themselves and found that, no matter how big the mammal (or the poop coming from that mammal), it took under fifteen seconds to go, from start to finish.

If you're someone who deals with chronic constipation, this may be shocking news, but as a mammal, that's about the time it should take you to go number two. If you have to spend a lot of time in the bathroom, straining and pushing, it's a glaring sign that your gut could use some help.

Next time you go to the bathroom, set a timer and see how long it takes you to feel fully emptied. Healthy poop typically comes right out in a minute or two, but anywhere from one to fifteen minutes is considered within the normal range. If you're way over that, it's time for a gut overhaul.

Note: When you're timing your poop, make sure you're only including the time it takes you to actually poop, not the time you spend in the bathroom scrolling through Instagram until your legs go numb. On that note, it's a good idea to leave your phone out of the bathroom when you go. The bathroom shouldn't be a place for mindless scrolling—the stress associated with social media use or checking your work emails can actually make it harder for you to go.

KEEP A POOP JOURNAL

Just like a food journal, a poop journal can give you clues about how your diet or lifestyle may be affecting your gut health. When you track your poop, you can figure out what helps your digestive system function best and what doesn't. This also helps you quickly identify any changes in your bowel habits, which is often the first sign of a potential problem.

Keep track of the following:

- What does your poop look like (size, shape, and color)?
- How long did it take you to poop? Did you have to strain? Did you feel empty afterward?
- Did you have pain in your stomach or rectum when pooping?
- Was there any blood, mucus, or undigested material in your poop?
- What did you eat that day?
- On a scale of 1 to 10, how stressed did you feel?
- Did you exercise that day? If so, what type of exercise did you do?

Instead of using pen and paper, you can download poop-tracking apps like Cara Care, Bowelle, PCal, and Bowel Mover Pro for iOS. If you search "poop app" in your app store, you'll find several different options.

These apps were designed for people dealing with irritable bowel syndrome, but they're a great tool for anyone. You can track your pooping habits, stress levels, food, and other factors right in the app so you can easily identify connections and patterns that indicate a need for some changes.

#10

PEEK AT YOUR PEE

When it comes to your gut health, your pee is just as important as your poop—after all, everything is connected. The color of your urine gives big clues about how hydrated you are, and proper hydration ensures that you're properly digesting your food, that waste materials are able to move through your digestive tract, and that your gut (and the rest of your body) is getting the nutrients it needs to function best.

Next time you go to the bathroom, peek in the toilet and check the color of your pee. If it's pale yellow to lemonade-colored, your body is hydrated and happy. If your pee looks more like light beer or amber ale, you're slightly to moderately dehydrated. If your pee is burnt orange to brownish in color, you're severely dehydrated, and it's beyond time to drink more water and electrolytes.

You should also pay attention to urinary frequency. Most people pee between six and eight times per day, but that can go up to ten if you're drinking a lot of water. If you're peeing a lot less than that, it's a good sign you're dehydrated. If you're peeing a lot more, it can be a sign of irritable bowel syndrome or gastroenteritis, especially if frequent urination is combined with any gastrointestinal distress.

#11

SMELL YOUR BREATH

This smell test isn't about your poop; it's about your breath. Chronic bad breath, officially referred to as halitosis, is often caused by bacteria and other microbes that live in your mouth. But if your oral care is on point and you still have bad breath that won't go away no matter what you do, it can be a sign that your gut flora is off.

Bad breath is often a sign of an overgrowth of *H. pylori*, but it goes hand in hand with constipation too. When you're not pooping regularly, the waste in your body can sit stagnant and back up in your system. Having an imbalanced gut can also make you more susceptible to health conditions like kidney problems and uncontrolled diabetes, which can also cause bad breath.

Often, when you have bad breath, you also have a bad taste in your mouth that's a pretty good indicator. But that's not always the case. To check your breath, you can breathe into your hand when it's cupped over your mouth or lick the inside of your wrist and then give it a quick sniff. If it smells unpleasant, it may be time for a gut overhaul. Mints and chewing gum may work temporarily, but the long-term solution is balancing your gut health.

#12

SNIFF YOUR PITS

Just as bad breath can be a sign of an unhealthy gut, so can unusual body odor. While lots of body odor is created on the skin—when bacteria come into contact with sweat, salt, sugar, and/or waste products—it can come from your gut too.

Your body uses things like stinky armpits to communicate messages to you about your health. If you suddenly smell different or you notice that you have an unusual amount of body odor compared to your activity level (you're just sitting on the couch watching *Netflix* rather than running), it's a pretty sure sign that something's off in your digestive tract.

Poor digestion and an imbalance in the gut can create a buildup of partially digested food and smelly by-products, like ammonia, sulfur compounds (the same compounds that give broccoli its characteristic scent), and/or trimethylamine, an ammonia-like compound that's been described as smelling like urine or rotten eggs.

Eating a lot of processed foods and foods high in sugar also increase body odor. These foods cause imbalances in the gut. They feed bad bacteria that give off toxic by-products that are often excreted through your skin.

Leaky gut (also known as intestinal permeability), a digestive condition in which the intestinal lining becomes permeable and bacteria and toxins are able to travel through it into the bloodstream, can also lead to widespread inflammation. This can cause a variety of problems, including hormone imbalances (like estrogen dominance) and autoimmune disorders that cause digestive issues, bad breath, and body odor. Stress, which is largely regulated by your gut, can also increase body odor.

#13

OPEN UP AND SAY "AHHHH"

You might not pay much attention to your tongue, but it's an important part of your digestive system—and it gives you a lot of clues about the state of your gut. If your tongue has a thick, white coating, it's a sign that your digestion is off or that you have a systemic candida (yeast) infection. You may also notice fatigue, joint pain, and frequent sinus infections along with the white coating.

White or gray patches may also indicate leukoplakia, which can be a sign that your diet is not up to par (although it can indicate other health conditions too). When your digestive system is overburdened—which usually happens when you eat a lot of refined carbohydrates or sugary foods—bacteria builds up on your tongue, leaving you with a bad taste in the morning.

Here are some other things your tongue can tell you:

- Redness = deficiency in folic acid, B_{12}, or iron
- Blue or purple = poor oxygen circulation (lung problems or kidney disease)
- Rough, dry, and cracked = dehydration
- Black and hairy looking = yeast infection, diabetes, or poor oral hygiene; may also be a side effect of cancer treatment
- Webbed or striped = chronic condition called oral lichen planus (autoimmunity that can be connected to your gut)
- Ridges = tongue inflammation or teeth pressing into your tongue while you sleep
- Bumps = canker sores and/or herpes

Your tongue should be pink with small bumps or nodules called papillae. If you see anything different, it's time to change what you're doing or go see your doctor.

#14

DO A SPIT TEST

A spit test can help determine if you have an overgrowth of yeast, fungus, or candida in your body. Keep in mind that this isn't a scientific test, but anecdotal evidence shows that it can be a good baseline for determining if you need to do some yeast cleansing or a candida diet. If you have a positive spit test, make an appointment with your functional medicine doctor (a doctor who uses an individualized approach and specializes in identifying and addressing the root cause of symptoms and/or disease) or a naturopath for a real candida test.

Here's how to do it:

1. As soon as you wake up—before you eat, drink, or brush your teeth—fill a clear glass with room-temperature water.
2. Gather a dime-sized amount of saliva and spit gently into the glass of water.
3. Let your saliva sit in the water for forty-five minutes.
4. After forty-five minutes, check for: stringy pieces coming down from the top of the water, cloudy specks suspended in the water, and/or cloudy saliva sitting in the bottom of the cup. These indicate the presence of candida and/or yeast.

Keep in mind that dairy consumption and dehydration can mess with your test results. Make sure you eliminate all dairy and drink the equivalent of half your body weight in ounces of water during the course of the day for at least a week before you do your spit test. If you're 200 pounds, that means 100 ounces of water.

"BEET" YOUR DIGESTIVE TRACT

The beet test is a simple way to check your transit time—how quickly food moves through your digestive tract. The average transit time is between thirty and forty hours, although anything between twelve and seventy-two hours is still considered normal. If your transit time is a lot shorter than that, it can indicate that food is moving too quickly through your bowels, not giving your body enough time to properly digest it and absorb the nutrients.

On the flip side, a much longer transit time can indicate that you have a sluggish bowel and that you're likely constipated. FYI: Even if you're going poop every day, you may still be constipated. The goal is to feel completely empty, without bloat or a full feeling in your stomach weighing you down.

Now, back to the beet test, which is simple. All you have to do is:

1. Eat a meal that contains beets. Raw beets are best, but you can eat cooked beets if you prefer. But try to avoid beet juice, since juice moves through your system faster than whole foods.
2. Write down the time and date you ate the beets.
3. Check the toilet every time you poop. When you see a red or purplish color, the beets have passed through.
4. Figure out how many hours it's been since you ate the beets. That's your current transit time.

Do this test a few times to figure out your average transit time. If the results are very different each time, talk with a functional medicine doctor or nutritionist to help figure out your next steps.

BUBBLE UP SOME BAKING SODA

Many people think acid reflux occurs as a result of too much stomach acid, but it's actually the exact opposite—a sign of too *little* stomach acid. Low stomach acid can also cause excessive burping or bloating after you eat and a heavy, dragging feeling in your stomach that doesn't seem to go away no matter what you do. If you think you might have stomach acid problems, there are a couple of easy tests that you can do right at home.

One of the quickest is the baking soda test. When baking soda comes into contact with stomach acid, it creates carbon dioxide gas as a by-product. The gas bubbles up in your stomach, making you feel like you have to burp.

To do the test, combine 1 cup of filtered water with $\frac{1}{4}$ teaspoon of baking soda and drink it down first thing in the morning on an empty stomach. If you haven't burped within two to three minutes of drinking the baking soda mixture, it's likely that you have low stomach acid.

Of course, this isn't a scientific test, but it can give you clues about where your gut stands. For best results, do the test on five consecutive mornings to see how the data compares. Keep in mind that this is a short-term test; it's not recommended to drink baking soda regularly.

#17

FEEL THE BETAINE HCl BURN

Betaine HCl is a supplemental form of hydrochloric acid or stomach acid. If you have normal levels of stomach acid and you take one of these supplements, you should feel a warm sensation in your stomach. That's because you're adding more stomach acid to the adequate levels you already have. If you have low stomach acid, it takes more than one to build up to a level where you feel that warmth.

To do the test, purchase a high-quality betaine HCl supplement with 650 to 750 milligrams per capsule. Some good options are:

- Designs for Health Betaine HCl
- Klaire Labs Betaine HCl
- Integrative Therapeutics Betaine HCl

On day one, take one capsule before a large meal. On day two, take two capsules before a large meal. On day three, take three capsules before a large meal. Repeat this three-capsule regimen for up to ten days until you feel warmth in your stomach after taking the supplements. The more supplements you have to take, the more likely you are to have low stomach acid.

If you do have low stomach acid, you can stay on the supplements to help correct the issue or you can make some other lifestyle changes, like taking apple cider vinegar, to help boost your levels.

If you have stomach ulcers, or a history of stomach ulcers, don't do the betaine HCl test.

SEE IF YOU'RE SENSITIVE

There's some controversy about whether or not food sensitivity tests are accurate, but even if they miss a few things, they provide a good baseline of what your body may be reacting to so you can start investigating whether or not you have a true food sensitivity.

The best way to identify food sensitivities is with a proper elimination diet, but if you find it hard to commit to one, you can also do a blood test to help guide an elimination diet. Food sensitivity tests are different from food allergy tests, although both measure immunoglobulins, which are antibodies created by your immune system.

It's important to note that a true food allergy produces an immune system response that could be life-threatening, depending on how serious your allergy is. A food sensitivity or intolerance causes a reaction that's triggered by your digestive system. Most doctors and allergists order true food allergy tests, but you can order food intolerance tests online and have them shipped right to your home. Typically, they involve pricking your finger, collecting a blood sample on a card, and then sending the sample to a lab to receive your results. You can order through a test through these companies:

- Everlywell.com
- HealthLabs.com
- TestMyAllergy.com
- AllergyTest.co

When you receive your results, try to avoid eating anything that comes up as a moderate to severe allergy for at least a month and see if that leads to any improvements in your symptoms or overall health. Of course, these tests aren't a substitute for a doctor's visit, and if you think you have a true food allergy, make an appointment to see your healthcare provider.

#19

SEARCH FOR HIDDEN INFECTIONS

The problem with gut infections is that they can be stealthy and, as a result, difficult to diagnose. Pathogenic bacteria, viruses, and parasites are opportunistic, meaning they look for opportunities to hide in your gut and do a good job of causing a lingering infection.

Keep in mind that no single gut health test is 100 percent reliable. That being said, one of the most accurate and comprehensive tests for gut infections is called a PCR stool analysis.

Traditional stool testing uses visual detection under a microscope, but a PCR test looks at DNA to detect bacteria, parasites, and viruses that shouldn't be in your poop. Even if you've had a negative stool test in the past, a PCR test can give you different—and more accurate—results.

Looking for hidden infections is an especially good idea if you have lingering symptoms that no one's been able to explain. Maybe all of your lab results have come back normal or you've been told time and time again that it's all in your head. There's a good chance that it's not all in your head, but actually in your gut.

#20

TEST YOUR OWN POOP

Gone are the days when you had to go to the doctor's office for every health test you wanted to take. Now you can test your own poop, right at home. Okay, so maybe that doesn't sound totally appealing, but an at-home stool test can give you lots of clues about your gut health, like:

- How well you're digesting your food
- Bacteria, yeast, and parasites that may be present
- Inflammation
- Immune function

And luckily, you don't have to actually test your poop yourself. Order a kit online and then follow the instructions to collect a sample and send it back to a lab for testing. Instructions vary, but typically you'll use a cotton swab to collect a small stool sample off your toilet paper after you go number two—easy-peasy.

There are all kinds of stool tests you can do at home, but some of the most popular are from:

- Viome
- Walk-In Lab
- Thryve

Some stool tests come with recommendations to follow based on your results, but you can also bring your results to a functional medicine doctor or a nutritionist to help you develop a comprehensive gut health plan.

BOOST YOUR VITAMIN D

All of the vitamins are important, but vitamin D should probably be in a class of its own. Vitamin D helps your body absorb calcium and maintain normal levels of calcium and phosphorus, which keeps your bones strong. But vitamin D also plays a crucial role in your gut health.

Vitamin D deficiency, or even a suboptimal level of vitamin D—meaning you're not technically deficient, but your levels are still kind of low—has been shown to promote gut inflammation, which can lead to bacterial imbalance, even if you're otherwise healthy. Vitamin D deficiency can also weaken the lining of your intestines, which can make you more susceptible to leaky gut.

Vitamin D deficiency is also connected to lowered production of defensins, antimicrobial molecules that are part of your immune system and essential to the proper balance of bacteria in your gut.

There's evidence that many people with inflammatory bowel diseases and autoimmune diseases have a vitamin D deficiency or low levels of vitamin D.

If you're having chronic health problems or gut issues—or even if you're not—it's important to know your vitamin D status. Vitamin D deficiency can be super-sneaky, but you can get your levels measured with a simple blood test. You can even order your own test kit to do at home.

While conventional medicine calls vitamin D levels of 20ng/mL normal, functional medicine (a systems based medical approach that identifies how and why symptoms and illness occur and then works to address individual causes to restore optimal health) practitioners like to see these levels closer to 50ng/mL for optimal health. If you get your vitamin D levels tested and they're low, work with a practitioner to find a high-quality vitamin D supplement that can help get your levels back to normal.

GO BIG ON YOUR B$_{12}$

Your gut and vitamin B$_{12}$ have a synergistic relationship. Vitamin B$_{12}$ plays an important role in balancing your gut bacteria and warding off gut inflammation. On the flip side, your gut (meaning your stomach and small intestine, in this case), need to be functioning optimally in order to absorb enough vitamin B$_{12}$.

Basically, your gut needs vitamin B$_{12}$ to function properly, but if your gut isn't functioning properly, you can't absorb the B$_{12}$ you need. That's a conundrum.

In addition to digestive issues like diarrhea, abdominal cramps, and nausea, some signs of vitamin B$_{12}$ deficiency include:

- Fatigue and/or low energy
- Muscle aches
- Muscle weakness
- Shortness of breath
- Dizziness/lightheadedness
- Loss of appetite
- Brain fog
- Poor concentration
- Memory loss
- Mood changes, depression, and/or anxiety
- Numbness and tingling in the hands or feet
- Heart palpitations

If you don't want to visit your doctor for a vitamin B$_{12}$ test, you can order a home test kit from labs like Everlywell. After collecting a blood sample (all you have to do is prick your finger), mail the sample in and wait for the results to find out your B$_{12}$ levels.

#23

BE B$_{12}$ SAVVY

Here's a crazy thing about vitamin B$_{12}$: It's possible to have a deficiency even if your blood levels are normal or high. This is called a functional B$_{12}$ deficiency, and it happens when you have enough vitamin B$_{12}$ circulating in your blood, but your body isn't able to use the nutrient. This is similar to how insulin resistance works—you have enough insulin in the blood, but your cells can't use it.

This happens for several reasons, but two of the most common are gut issues and/or a glutathione deficiency. It's important to catch this because an undiagnosed vitamin B$_{12}$ deficiency can eventually cause permanent nerve damage and other issues that can be prevented with early intervention.

If your blood results come back with a high or normal vitamin B$_{12}$, but you have all of the symptoms of a vitamin B$_{12}$ deficiency, ask your doctor for a methylmalonic acid (MMA) test and a homocysteine test. High levels of both of these can point to a vitamin B$_{12}$ deficiency, even if your vitamin B$_{12}$ levels are normal.

ADD SOME A TO YOUR LIFE

Vitamin A is often called the vision vitamin because it's intricately connected to good eye health, but it's extremely important for your gut health too. The short explanation is that vitamin A maintains the immune system in your gut and controls T cells, B cells, and dendritic cells, which are sent out in response to potential health threats.

Vitamin A also regulates the intestinal epithelium, the lining of both your small and large intestines that plays a role in the creation of the mucus layer that covers everything. If your vitamin A levels are low, it leaves your gut susceptible to infection and negatively affects the integrity of your gut lining, which can eventually lead to leaky gut.

The official way to get your vitamin A status is to ask your doctor for a blood test or a retinol test, but you can also do a self-check at home to see if you have the symptoms of a vitamin A deficiency, which include:

- Acne
- Skin infections that won't go away
- Dry, patchy skin
- Throat infections, canker sores, or mouth ulcers
- Dandruff
- Dry hair and/or hair breakage
- Poor and/or declining night vision
- Sore eyelids

If you have a couple of (or all of) these symptoms, it might be a sign that you need a little more vitamin A in your life to reach optimal gut health.

#25

MEET THE MASTER (ANTIOXIDANT)

Glutathione is often called "the master antioxidant" because it's important for every function in your body. It's critical to immune function and natural detoxification, and without it, your detox organs like your kidneys and liver can't do their jobs properly. And if your detox pathways aren't working as they should, it can lead to a buildup of toxins and free radicals and cause chronic inflammation.

Glutathione also helps your body use vitamin B_{12}, so if you don't have enough, it can lead to a vitamin B_{12} deficiency, which can then lead to gut dysbiosis and gut inflammation.

Because of that, glutathione deficiency has been connected to many chronic conditions, including chronic fatigue syndrome, heart disease, generalized anxiety disorder, cancer, chronic infections, autoimmune disease, diabetes, autism, Alzheimer's disease, Parkinson's disease, arthritis, asthma, kidney problems, and liver disease.

Your body creates its own glutathione, but things like poor diet, too much stress, emotional distress, too much strenuous exercise, exposure to toxic chemicals, pollution, and radiation can all deplete glutathione and interfere with your body's ability to produce it.

The symptoms of a glutathione deficiency include:

- Fatigue
- Lack of energy
- Pain in your muscles and/or joints
- Poor concentration
- Sleep disturbances
- Frequent sickness and/or infections

If you suspect you have a glutathione deficiency, or you've gotten your vitamin B_{12} levels checked and they're high but you still feel like something is off, ask your doctor for an RBC glutathione test. This test measures the amount of glutathione in your red blood cells.

IRON OUT YOUR IRON

Most of the healthy bacteria in your gut require iron to grow and multiply. If you don't have enough iron, it can lead to bacterial imbalances and gut dysbiosis. Iron also helps your gut produce short-chain fatty acids, which further fuel your good bacteria and act as a source of energy for you.

Interestingly, a healthy gut is also necessary to properly absorb iron. If your gut is inflamed and teeming with bad bacteria, you can't properly absorb iron. And if you can't properly absorb iron, it's hard to get your gut back in balance. The good news is that incorporating several different gut health hacks into your life can help reduce inflammation and put your gut on track to better iron absorption.

But since iron can accumulate in your body and lead to toxicity, you don't want to supplement with iron unless you know for sure that you're deficient. To find out, ask your doctor for a serum iron test, a transferrin test, and a ferritin test. These tests can tell you your current iron levels and give you clues as to whether or not your body has a problem storing iron.

Iron test kits available online or through pharmacies allow you to test your own levels with a kit that comes right to your home.

#27

MANAGE YOUR MAGNESIUM

Magnesium is the fourth most abundant mineral in your body. But over the past few years, health experts have noticed an alarming trend: More than 60 percent of Americans don't get enough magnesium daily, and as a result, magnesium deficiency is quickly becoming a public health crisis. One of the best ways to determine whether you're at risk of magnesium deficiency (or if you have one already) is to assess your risk factors.

Major risk factors are:

- High soda intake
- Consumption of lots of processed foods
- Use (or prior use) of diuretics and/or antacids
- Diabetes, heart disease, and metabolic syndrome

Minor risk factors are:

- Alcohol consumption
- Use or prior use of oral contraceptives and/or antibiotics
- BMI (body mass index) greater than 30
- Osteoporosis

If you do (or have done) a couple of these things, it's likely you need some more magnesium in your life. If you've experienced leg cramps, trouble sleeping, fibromyalgia (widespread pain), and chronic fatigue, those are also telltale signs of a magnesium deficiency.

But what does this have to do with gut health? Magnesium ensures your muscles are working correctly, and that includes the muscles in your digestive tract. If they're not working correctly, you can get constipated quickly. Magnesium also helps you sleep and plays a part in how your body handles stress—two things that are vital for gut health.

#28

AVOID HEAVY METALS

Your gut bacteria are the first line of defense against heavy metals. They play a few major roles in protecting you:

- They act as a physical barrier, blocking absorption through the digestive tract.
- They interfere with the metabolism of heavy metals.
- They change the pH balance and concentration of enzymes and proteins that break down heavy metals to prevent absorption.

But by doing all this, your gut bacteria put themselves in the line of fire, so to speak. By protecting you, some of them end up dying off, and, as a result, the balance of bacteria in your gut changes, and you're left more susceptible to the symptoms and chronic diseases associated with poor gut health.

Rather than relying on your gut bacteria to protect you from heavy metals, it's a better idea to avoid them as much as possible while also properly supporting your gut function. It's also a good idea to find out if you're dealing with a heavy metal toxicity so you can take steps to get rid of the heavy metals that are in your system already.

You can order an at-home heavy metal test that assesses your levels of arsenic, bromine, cadmium, and mercury. It also measures your selenium levels, since selenium helps counteract the effects of heavy metals. If your heavy metals are high and your selenium level is low, it may be a sign that your gut is being negatively affected. If you discover that you have some heavy metal toxicity, part of your gut health protocol should be getting rid of that heavy metal buildup.

HALT HIGH HISTAMINE

Do you:

- Get diarrhea a lot?
- Have regular headaches?
- Experience frequent anxiety?
- Get an itchy tongue or runny nose when you eat certain foods, like bananas or avocados?
- Have a flushed face after you drink red wine?

If you answered yes to several of these questions, it's possible you have a histamine intolerance. Histamine is a chemical compound that's naturally produced by your body. It has several roles, including:

- Sending signals back and forth from your brain
- Stimulating the release of stomach acid to help digestion
- Playing a role in your immune response when you get injured or have an allergic reaction

Normally, histamine levels rise and fall, but if you have a histamine intolerance, it means that your levels of histamine have gotten too high. Histamine intolerance is closely linked to leaky gut and small intestinal bacterial overgrowth (SIBO).

To test if you have a histamine intolerance, you can do a DAO trial. DAO, or diamine oxidase, is an enzyme that breaks histamine down in your gut. Sometimes, when you have a histamine intolerance, you don't have adequate levels of DAO, and that causes the buildup.

The test is easy to do: Take a DAO supplement at each meal for two weeks and see if your symptoms improve. If they do, it's likely that you have a histamine intolerance, and you can move on to a low-histamine diet and working on fixing your gut to correct the problem.

#30

GET A THYROID WORKUP

There's an intricate connection between your thyroid and your gut. The two communicate with each other through something called the thyroid-gut axis. When your gut isn't healthy, your thyroid isn't healthy, and vice versa.

Because of this, Graves' disease and Hashimoto's thyroiditis, which are the most common autoimmune thyroid diseases, often occur hand in hand with celiac disease and gluten and/or wheat intolerance. That's why getting your thyroid checked can give you important clues about your gut health as well.

When you have your physical or regular checkup, most doctors only check the levels of TSH, or thyroid stimulating hormone. TSH is the hormone that's made by your pituitary gland. When levels go up, it tells your thyroid to make thyroid hormones and release them into your blood.

If your levels of TSH are normal, your doctor may make a determination that your thyroid is functioning normally. But in reality, your thyroid antibodies (TPO and TG) may be elevated and attacking your thyroid for several years before your TSH levels register as abnormal.

When you go for a thyroid checkup, ask your doctor to order values for:

- TPO
- TG
- TSH
- Free T3
- Free T4

All of these values together can give you a complete picture of the state of your thyroid and the state of your gut.

PINCH YOUR ARM

Your skin contains compounds like collagen and elastin that keep it springy and help it bounce back into place. This is called skin turgor. When you pinch your skin, it should return back to normal within one or two seconds. If it doesn't, that's a pretty good sign you're dehydrated. And dehydration can lead to imbalanced gut bacteria, constipation, slowed digestion, and bloating.

To do the pinch test, pinch the skin on your arm or stomach for a few seconds and then let go. If it bounces right back within a second or two, your skin turgor is normal. If it takes longer than that, there's likely some dehydration going on—and the longer it takes to spring back into place, the more dehydrated you are.

Note: This isn't the most accurate test for people over the age of sixty-five, as skin naturally loses elasticity as you get older. If you're older, skin takes about twenty seconds, on average, to return to normal even if you aren't dehydrated.

TAKE A BREATH (TEST)

If you're dealing with constant bloating, burping, stomach cramps, constipation/diarrhea, heartburn, nausea, headaches, and fatigue, it's possible that you have small intestinal bacterial overgrowth, or SIBO.

But what is it? Normally, bacteria live in your large intestine. But sometimes, thanks to things like low stomach acid, use of oral contraceptives, frequent antibiotic use, prior bowel surgery, or intestinal diseases (like Crohn's disease and irritable bowel syndrome), those bacteria can migrate to your small intestine, where they don't belong.

A SIBO breath test, officially called a lactulose breath test, measures how the bacteria in your gut are functioning over a three-hour period. It can give clues about whether or not the bacteria in your gut is where it belongs. On a basic level, this is how it works:

- You drink a solution of lactulose, a man-made sugar that humans can't digest but that small intestinal bacteria thrive on. You may experience some bloating, gas, or diarrhea.
- After drinking the solution, you or your doctor will collect a breath sample utilizing a tube and straw method. Your breath sample will be sent to the lab where hydrogen and methane, two gases created as a by-product of bacteria fermenting the lactulose, will be measured.
- The amount and type of gas present tells you or your doctor where bacteria are residing in your GI tract and whether or not there's an overproduction of gas.

You can purchase an at-home SIBO test kit from Life Extension or Metabolic Solutions. The results will let you know whether or not it's necessary to follow a SIBO treatment protocol, which may involve a combination of antibiotics and various gut health hacks.

#33

SCRUTINIZE YOUR STRESS LEVELS

Stress and your gut go together like peanut butter and jelly. Okay, maybe that isn't the best simile, but the point is that your stress levels and your gut health are completely tied together. If you're stressed out, your gut is stressed out. And if your gut is stressed out, it can actually affect the way that your body balances its stress hormones.

You probably don't need a test to tell you if you're stressed or not, but a test *can* tell you if your stress is affecting your body on a physiological level. Everyone reacts and responds to stress differently, so if you're experiencing high levels of stress but managing it well, your hormones may be normal. On the flip side, if stress has completely overwhelmed you, it's likely that your hormones are out of whack and your stress is a major contributor to any gut problems.

Fortunately, there's an easy way to check this at home. The Sleep and Stress Test from Everlywell measures cortisol, cortisone, and melatonin through easy-to-collect urine samples. The results will tell you if your stress hormones are high and/or your sleep hormones are low or if they follow an abnormal pattern. Based on these results, you'll know if you need to prioritize stress relief and hormone balancing as part of your gut health protocol.

#34

SCAN YOUR SKIN

Your gut and skin are connected through a pathway called the gut-skin axis. Your skin has several major roles, including protection from the outside world, water retention, and temperature regulation. It's constantly regenerating itself through several different processes that are ultimately controlled by your gut.

If you're struggling with skin issues, you've probably heard someone say that manifestations on the skin often come from inside. And while the unsolicited advice may have annoyed you at the time, it's actually true. Studies show that people with eczema, acne, and rosacea are up to ten times more likely to have gut issues, while 34 percent of people with irritable bowel syndrome also have problems with their skin.

Your skin isn't able to maintain homeostasis, or balance, if your gut isn't functioning properly. So if you have chronic skin issues, like acne, eczema, or psoriasis, or constantly itchy skin or unexplained bumps that just don't seem to go away no matter what you do, it's likely that you have a gut issue going on underneath the surface.

#35

CONTEMPLATE YOUR POOP SCHEDULE

When it comes to bathroom frequency, there's no "normal" number of times you should go. For some people, going three times a day is a regular part of life, but for others, that can signal that something is wrong.

Poop frequency only becomes a problem if your stools are abnormal or they're accompanied by uncomfortable symptoms like gas, bloating, and stomach pain. Or if the need to go to the bathroom is so urgent that you often feel like you're on the verge of having an accident. Changes in normal frequency can also signal an issue. If you generally poop once a day, and suddenly you're going three or four times, something else is likely going on underneath the surface.

When you're assessing your gut health, figure out what's normal for you and pay attention to any changes in that routine. Of course, what you're eating and the amount of exercise you're getting can play a role in poop frequency, but if you're suddenly going to the bathroom much more than you used to, and you don't feel good overall, that's a sign of poor gut health.

#36

CURB YOUR SUGAR CRAVINGS

Sugar cravings are often deemed a "sweet tooth," but most of the time, they originate in your gut. When you have too much bad bacteria or an overgrowth of candida, a yeast (or fungus), it can trigger an out-of-control desire for sweets. These bad bugs actually take over neurotransmitters in your gut, brain, and vagus nerve and send out signals that make you crave sugary, carbohydrate-rich foods until you finally give in.

The sugar then feeds the yeast and bad bacteria, they continue to grow, and this cycle repeats on an endless loop. In other words, gut bacteria are really the problem and the solution here. This is also the reason why willpower and self-discipline don't always work. The bugs in your gut are screaming for sugar, and they get louder and louder until you give in.

If your sugar cravings are out of control, meaning you constantly crave sugar or you can't control your sugar portions once you get a taste of something sweet, it's a good sign that your gut is out of whack. And the more you give in to those cravings, the more imbalanced things become.

#37

CONSULT THE SCALE

If you're doing everything "right," and your weight is still steadily creeping upward, it may be a sign that something's not quite right in your gut. In a 2009 study published in *Nature*, researchers looked at the gut microbiome of identical twins and found that the lower the bacterial diversity in the gut (meaning fewer strains of different types of bacteria), the more likely you are to be overweight and/or gain weight.

Weighing yourself every morning can be a good way to keep track of whether or not your gut is functioning properly. While the number on the scale isn't the best measure of your overall health, it can allow you to monitor changes that seem abnormal. Small fluctuations—a couple of pounds up and down—are normal, but if you notice that your weight is steadily creeping upward, especially if it's combined with bloating and/or constipation, that's a good sign that something is going on underneath the surface.

It's helpful to weigh yourself at the same time every day (usually the first thing in the morning) and then log that number. Try not to get caught up in the actual number, but rather use it as a reference point as to what your "normal" is. If you have a history of disordered eating or an unhealthy relationship with the number on the scale, you don't actually have to weigh yourself, but pay attention to any unexplained weight changes by the way your clothes fit or the way you feel in general.

Make sure you're being honest with yourself. If you've been sitting for fourteen hours a day and eating more chips than usual, that weight gain can be pretty easily explained.

LOG YOUR HEADACHES

For reasons that aren't totally clear, migraines and headaches are often connected to poor gut health. In a study that was published in *The Journal of Headache and Pain* in 2020, researchers pointed out that people who frequently get migraines or headaches also have a higher chance of being diagnosed with irritable bowel syndrome (IBS) and Crohn's disease. The researchers speculated that the inflammation associated with the digestive conditions also resulted in the head pain. The researchers also connected high levels of *H. pylori* to headaches and migraines and found that when that bacterial imbalance in the gut was corrected, patients' headaches decreased.

Other studies suggest that in addition to the inflammation and inflammatory factors, there's a bidirectional (two-way) relationship between the gut and the brain that's also influenced by bacteria in your gut, stress hormones, the serotonin produced by your gut, and the food you're eating.

Every time you get a headache, write it down somewhere (a journal or planner is a great way to keep it all in one place) and rate the intensity on a scale of one to ten. If you're experiencing headaches more often than not, all signs point to gut health.

#39

CHECK YOUR BLOAT

Occasional bloating is normal. The average person produces between 500 and 1,500 milliliters of gas per day, which is an amount that could fill up a 2-liter bottle of soda. If you let it out, either by burping or farting, then you're less likely to bloat. But if you hold it in, it can result in abdominal bloating and pain.

Bloating can be caused by things that are pretty easy to correct:

- Eating too fast
- Not chewing enough
- Drinking carbonated beverages
- Not drinking enough water
- Eating oversized portions

But bloating can also be caused by digestive conditions and/or things that don't agree with you or support optimal gut health. These are a little harder to balance out:

- Irritable bowel syndrome
- Celiac disease
- Lactose intolerance
- Constipation
- Gastroesophageal reflux disease (GERD)
- GI infections, like SIBO and/or *H. pylori*
- Food intolerances
- Excess stress

This isn't really a test per se, but pay attention to how you feel after you eat and how you feel when you wake up in the morning. If you're bloated all the time and your stomach never feels emptied, there may be a gut issue going on underneath the surface.

MIND THOSE MOOD SWINGS

If you're always anxious, depressed, irritable, and/or impatient, or you experience regular mood swings—first you're up, then all of a sudden you're crying—it may be a sign that there's something going on in your gut.

Hormones made in your gut, classified as gut peptides, control the signaling between your gut and your brain (and vice versa). If these hormone levels are thrown off by things like poor diet, gut inflammation, or too much stress, to name a few, it can cause anxiety and other mood issues. If you have gut issues, it can also affect the way you absorb certain vitamins and minerals. Not getting enough of certain nutrients can lead to deficiencies connected to low mood, anxiety, and/or mood swings.

A mood tracker is a simple way to monitor your moods so that you can see what's going on with your mental health (and your gut health too). A simple way to keep a mood tracker is to have a journal or planner where you write down how you feel every day. These can be simple statements, like "I feel anxious" or "I feel happy." You can also rate your feelings on a scale of one to ten, since emotions and moods don't always feel the same.

If you keep a mood and food tracker at the same time, you may be able to make connections between what you're eating and how you're feeling. For example, on days where you eat a lot of sugar or processed foods, you may notice that you feel more anxious than usual. Keep track of these connections so you know how foods affect you.

Chapter 2

CHANGE YOUR DIET AND EATING PATTERNS

Although a lot of factors are involved in your gut health, the food you eat (and how you eat it) is the foundation that everything else is built on. Everything you put in your mouth either feeds and supports your good bacteria and digestive fluids, like your stomach acid and digestive enzymes, or promotes the growth of bad bacteria and makes it harder for good bacteria to thrive. And when bad bacteria outweigh the good—a situation that's called an unbalanced gut microbiome—you're susceptible to gut issues. Your diet is the key to maintaining the integrity of your intestinal lining.

A healthy gut has a tight intestinal lining that's very discerning and only allows nanoparticles to pass through. However, when you eat foods that promote inflammation and intestinal damage, it can cause gaps that allow bigger particles to travel into your blood, a condition called "leaky gut." When this happens, the bigger particles that aren't supposed to be there can trigger chronic inflammatory and allergic reactions that lead to a whole array of symptoms.

The hacks in this chapter will teach you how to eat in a way that supports your gut health, from balancing your microbiome to preventing and/or reversing leaky gut. You will also learn the best foods to eat to keep your digestion regular, so you can have consistent bowel movements. And if you've ever experienced constipation, you know that pooping is the key to feeling your best.

THROW AWAY PROCESSED FOODS

If there's nothing else you do for your gut, do this: Get processed foods out of your diet. Processed foods are the number one contributor to gut dysbiosis. They're often full of unhealthy fats, white sugar, and artificial ingredients and almost completely devoid of fiber. This combination not only starves good bacteria, it allows bad bacteria to run rampant, leaving you bloated, gassy, constipated, and just plain cranky.

There's no doubt that processed foods are convenient, but because they mess up your gut, they're connected to all sorts of related health problems, like weight gain, obesity, and noncommunicable diseases like cancer, heart disease, nonalcoholic fatty liver disease, and diabetes (to name a few of the big ones).

The foods that are at fault are not just obviously unhealthy processed foods like macaroni and cheese and frozen pizza; they're *all* types of processed foods, even the gluten-free or low-sugar ones. That includes:

- Cereal
- Potato chips/tortilla chips
- Bread
- Granola bars
- Crackers
- Cookies
- Frozen dinners

Keep in mind that there are different levels of processing. While frozen vegetables are technically processed, they're still a healthy choice. The goal is to avoid ready-to-eat, convenience foods that lack proper nutrition and the fiber your gut needs.

FILL 'ER UP ON FIBER

On average, Americans eat about 16 grams of fiber per day, which isn't nearly enough. The current recommendation for women is 25 grams daily, while men need about 38 grams per day.

Low fiber intake can cause gut problems like constipation and decreased bacterial diversity—or not enough of different kinds of bacteria in your gut. Falling short on your fiber can also create long-term health problems, like an increased risk of heart disease and cancer. And since many of the most nutrient-dense foods are the ones that are highest in fiber, if you're not getting enough fiber, it's highly likely that you're low on other nutrients too.

If you think your fiber intake is low, the best way to boost your intake is to start adding a plant food to each of your meals. For example, you can throw some kale and spinach into your eggs in the morning or mix some chia seeds into your yogurt. Add a side of vegetables—any vegetables—to your lunch and eat a side salad with your dinner.

Some of the best sources of fiber are:

- Avocados
- Raspberries
- Lentils
- Artichokes
- Split peas
- Chickpeas
- Chia seeds
- Flaxseed

- Almonds
- Beets
- Broccoli
- Bananas
- Apples
- Beans
- Oats

#43

DOUBLE THE FIBER, DOUBLE THE GOOD

Fiber is a type of carbohydrate that your body cannot fully digest. There are two main types—soluble and insoluble—and both are found exclusively in plant foods. Your body handles each type of fiber differently, and, because of that, they play different roles in your body and in your health.

As its name implies, soluble fiber dissolves in water and then turns to gel in your digestive tract. It helps improve digestion and can normalize your cholesterol levels. Many soluble fibers, especially those that are fermentable, act as a prebiotic, or a source of food for the bacteria that naturally live in your gut. Foods rich in soluble fiber include: apples, apricots, beans, blueberries, broccoli, carrots, lentils, nuts, pears, and sweet potatoes.

Insoluble fiber doesn't dissolve in water, so it passes through your digestive system almost completely intact. When insoluble fiber goes through the digestive tract, it pulls water into your stool, which makes it softer and easier to pass. This effect is similar to bulk-forming laxatives and can help alleviate constipation and improve gut health and function. Foods rich in insoluble fiber include: avocados, beans, cauliflower, chia seeds, dark leafy greens, potatoes, and vegetable skins.

If you want to keep your gut in the best shape possible, it's important to get both types of fiber regularly. The best way is to make sure you're eating lots of different types of foods and adding more plants to your diet.

FEAST ON SOME FERMENTED FOODS

Fermentation, which is the breakdown of carbohydrates by bacteria and yeast, is the original form of food processing. The goal of fermentation was to increase the shelf life of foods before there was access to refrigeration. But since bacteria and yeast are used during the fermentation process, it also creates loads of probiotics in the food that make food more digestible, boost immune health, and improve gut health by promoting a healthy balance of bacteria.

While there's a lot of focus on supplements to give you the probiotics you need, researchers from an August 2016 report in *Functional Foods in Health and Disease* tested fermented foods like sauerkraut to see how many probiotics they actually contained. Even the smallest serving of sauerkraut tested (2 tablespoons) had one million colony-forming units, or CFUs.

Not only do fermented foods have high numbers of probiotics, they also contain a wide diversity, or different forms of probiotics.

A September 2018 study found that the probiotics in fermented foods also seem to be more resistant than supplements to the low pH of stomach acid. In other words, unlike some supplemental probiotics, they don't get killed in your stomach. Instead, they travel through all the way to your small intestine, where they can grow, multiply, and keep your gut healthy. Some fermented foods are:

- Sauerkraut (unpasteurized)
- Yogurt (with live active cultures)
- Cheese (with live active cultures)
- Pickles (naturally fermented)
- Kefir
- Miso
- Green olives
- Tempeh
- Natto
- Kombucha
- Kimchi

PUMP UP THE PREBIOTICS

When it comes to gut health, probiotics get a lot of attention, but prebiotics are just as important. Prebiotics are nondigestible fibers that feed the good bacteria in your gut. They include inulin, fructooligosaccharides, galactooligosaccharides, beta-glucans, pectins, and resistant starches.

When you eat foods that are high in any of these prebiotic fibers, you're giving the good bacteria the nourishment they need to grow and multiply. On the other hand, if you don't eat any prebiotic foods, you're starving your good bacteria of the food they need to survive.

This is why you often hear that plant foods are the best choices for gut health. Plant foods are the only sources of prebiotic fibers. Some prebiotic-rich foods include:

- Jerusalem artichokes
- Dandelion greens
- Asparagus
- Garlic
- Onions
- Leeks
- Bananas (especially if they aren't quite ripe yet)
- Plantains
- Seaweed
- Shiitake mushrooms
- Jicama
- Konjac root
- Burdock root
- Yacon root
- Raw, unpasteurized apple cider vinegar

Different types of foods and fibers feed different types of bacteria, so when you eat a variety of prebiotic foods, you increase your chances of having a highly diverse bacterial population in your gut—and that's a good thing.

SWAP YOUR COFFEE FOR CHICORY ROOT

Chicory coffee is a hot beverage that's made from the roots of the chicory plant, a woody perennial that's part of the dandelion family. Chicory has a high concentration of inulin, a fiber that acts as a prebiotic. Chicory is also rich in polyphenols, antioxidant compounds that act as prebiotics and help balance your gut ecosystem.

Coffee has potential health risks, mostly due to its caffeine, and as many people are sensitive to caffeine, there's an increasing demand for a caffeine-free substitute. That's where chicory root coffee comes in. It doesn't actually contain any coffee. It's made from chicory root that's been roasted, dried, and ground into a powder that you can mix with water or steamed milk to make a latte.

It doesn't taste exactly like coffee—let's be honest, there's no great caffeine-free substitute that comes close to the real thing. But a steaming mug of chicory root does provide that warm, comforting feeling that coffee is known for. And since you'll be doing something good for your gut, the trade-off is worth it.

Pro tip: Get a handheld frother and heat up some oat milk on the stove over low heat. Use your handheld frother to aerate the milk. Fill a mug with two-thirds chicory root coffee and fill the remaining one-third with the oat milk for an easy homemade latte.

#47

DRINK SOME MUSHROOMS

Medicinal mushrooms—like reishi, chaga, lion's mane, shiitake, cordyceps, and turkey tail—are earning a serious name for themselves in the health world, and for good reason. Manufacturers take the mushrooms, which are classified as macroscopic fungi, and turn them into extracts or powders that have powerful health benefits and have been used to treat skin diseases and support the nervous system.

Because medicinal mushrooms are rich in carbohydrates like beta-glucans, chitin, hemicellulose, and galactans, they're one of the strongest prebiotics you can get. When you add them to your diet, they may help stimulate the growth and reproduction of good bacteria in your gut, which can improve metabolic health and reduce inflammation. Medicinal mushrooms may also:

- Boost and support your immune system
- Prevent cancer
- Supply loads of antioxidants
- Improve blood pressure and circulation
- Lower cholesterol
- Fight off inflammation
- Improve cognition, memory, and concentration
- Boost energy

Lots of different types of mushroom powders are available. You can use them to make a healthier version of hot chocolate (many are mixed with cacao, another superfood that promotes the growth of good bacteria and reduces gut inflammation), mix them into coffee or tea, or blend them into your smoothies. You can even add them to soup broths and baked goods. They blend in easily, but do add an umami taste that many people really enjoy.

#48

SIP ON BLACK TEA

Green tea tends to get a lot of attention, but you should give black tea a little love too. Black tea is loaded with polyphenols, plant compounds that act as prebiotics in your gut and promote the growth of good bacteria. Black tea may also be able to positively change your gut in a way that contributes to weight loss and/or prevents weight gain.

Certain bacteria in your gut promote weight gain and obesity. If your gut is healthy, the number of these bacteria stays fairly low and you have an easier time maintaining a healthy weight. However, if the number of these bacteria grow, it can contribute to weight gain and make it difficult for you to lose weight, no matter what you do. That's because the bacteria in your gut can actually regulate the amount of fat you absorb. *Firmicutes* bacteria, which are categorized as obesogenic, promote weight gain, while *Bacteroidetes* promote lean body mass.

Researchers from UCLA did a study on how the compounds in black tea could affect the bacteria in your gut. They found that these compounds decrease *Firmicutes* (the kind that make you gain weight), while increasing *Bacteroidetes* (the kind that help you maintain a healthy weight).

The study also found that the polyphenols in black tea are too large to pass through the small intestines and into the blood. Because of this, they move to the large intestine, where bacteria feed on them, producing short-chain fatty acids (SCFAs) as a by-product. These fatty acids positively change the way you metabolize your food, contributing to weight loss and overall good health. So, if you want to keep your gut healthy, drink black tea a few times a week.

#49

CUT OUT SUGAR

There was a time when health professionals thought that sugar wasn't good for you simply because it was full of empty calories. But as more research around sugar is being done, it's become evident that the detrimental effects go beyond that. Eating a lot of sugar doesn't just add a lot of calories to your day; it also decreases the amount of good bacteria in your gut. Sugar also contributes to chronic inflammation, which decreases the diversity of your gut bacteria and hinders their function.

It also drives metabolic dysfunction, contributes to high blood sugar, high cholesterol, high blood pressure, fatty liver disease, weight gain, obesity, and chronic inflammation. It disrupts your brain chemistry, contributing to anxiety and depression. And it's addictive, so the more you eat, the more you want. Studies show that eating sugar lights up the same part of the brain that lights up when alcoholics have a drink, which increases your cravings and contributes to bingeing behavior. This doesn't mean that you have to avoid sugar forever, but if you're having gut problems, it's a good idea to avoid it until you're able to get things back in balance.

One of the worst types of sugar is high-fructose corn syrup, which is highly processed and contributes to lots of health problems, like metabolic syndrome, nonalcoholic fatty liver disease, and type 2 diabetes. If you can't limit all types of sugar, make sure you're at least avoiding this one as much as you can.

AVOID ARTIFICIAL SWEETENERS

Artificial sweeteners were invented for people who can't eat sugar, namely diabetics, or people who are trying to avoid taking in excess calories. They seem to provide the best of both worlds—a sweet taste without any of the carbs or calories. Genius, right? Not exactly.

In an animal study that was published in the scientific journal *Molecules*, researchers found that the six most common artificial sweeteners approved by the FDA are actually toxic to gut bacteria. When you consume these sweeteners, it's possible that they're contributing to a gut imbalance that can have a wide range of health effects and a negative effect on your metabolism. Another interesting finding from the study was that the artificial sweeteners actually contributed to glucose intolerance (poor blood sugar control)—the very thing they were invented to prevent.

The six approved artificial sweeteners are:

- Aspartame
- Sucralose
- Saccharine
- Neotame
- Advantame
- Acesulfame potassium or acesulfame-K

These sweeteners are commonly found in "diet" or "light" packaged foods and beverages or anything marketed as calorie-free. If you want to make sure your gut is in top shape, read labels diligently and avoid anything that contains any of these names in the ingredient list.

If you need a way to sweeten things up without the carbs or calories, stick to stevia or erythritol, a sugar alcohol that hasn't been shown to cause any digestive upset. Try not to get in the habit of using any type of calorie-free sweeteners regularly, though. Getting rid of your sweet craving is a better idea.

#51

CUE UP THE QUERCETIN

At some point in your life, someone has probably told you that "an apple a day keeps the doctor away." While you may have thought this was just a cute way of saying you should eat more fruits and vegetables, there's actually a lot of truth behind it.

Apples are rich in quercetin, an antioxidant that helps increase bacterial diversity in the gut. Quercetin also reduces inflammation, which contributes to leaky gut, and helps repair the intestinal lining, plugging up any holes or leaks.

Researchers from a 2019 study published in *Frontiers in Microbiology* found that apples are covered in diverse bacteria that populate your gut and contribute to a healthy microbiome. The researchers estimated that a single apple contains one hundred million different bacteria of many different species. Much of that bacteria are found in the core and seeds, but if you're not a core eater, you can get about ten million bacteria by eating the flesh and skin.

The researchers also noted that organic apples have more diverse bacteria than nonorganic apples. Organic apples also contain fewer pesticides that can damage your gut, so when you're eating your daily apple, it's best to go organic whenever possible.

You can also get quercetin in supplemental form or from other foods and herbs, like:

- Dill
- Cilantro
- Capers
- Tomatoes
- Kale
- Cranberries
- Raspberries
- Red grapes
- Cherries
- Radishes
- Red onions

MUNCH ON SOME MANGO

Mangoes are a juicy, tropical treat that have some serious gut health benefits too. In a 2018 study published in *Molecular Nutrition & Food Research*, researchers compared eating a mango to taking a similar amount of fiber in the form of a fiber supplement and found that the mango helped alleviate constipation better.

For the study, thirty-six adults with chronic constipation were split into two groups. One group ate 2 cups fresh mango (equivalent to one mango), and the other consumed 1 teaspoon psyllium husk, which provides 5 grams of fiber. The mango group experienced several positive benefits, like more frequent stools and better stool consistency and shape. They also had higher levels of short-chain fatty acids (SCFAs), which help improve bacterial diversity in the gut, and reduced markers of inflammation. The researchers attributed the difference to the mangoes' level of polyphenols—a class of antioxidants that help reduce inflammation and contribute to the balance of bacteria and other microorganisms in your gut.

In another study published in the *Journal of Nutrition*, researchers found that mango could actually counteract the gut bacteria–destroying effects of a bad diet. That doesn't mean that eating mango can take the place of eating well, but this fruit makes a welcome addition to any gut-friendly diet. Mangoes have also been shown to help regulate blood sugar and make it easier for you to lose weight—wins all around.

In addition to buying them fresh, you can buy frozen mango chunks and make a smoothie with a slightly green banana (for added resistant starch) or stir them into yogurt for a real gut-boosting treat.

EAT YOUR BANANAS GREEN(ISH)

Have you ever eaten a green(ish) banana that wasn't quite ripe and felt chalkiness in your mouth? That's resistant starch, a type of carbohydrate that can't be broken down by your stomach and small intestine. That's why it's called *resistant* starch—it's resistant to digestion.

Resistant starch travels through your digestive system to your large intestine (specifically your colon), where it feeds the good bacteria in your gut. As the bacteria eat the resistant starch, it increases their numbers and promotes the growth of different types of good bacteria. This creates a balanced and diverse intestinal ecosystem that contributes to a healthy gut.

When the bacteria are done feeding on the resistant starch, they create by-products called short-chain fatty acids, or SCFAs. The most notable of these SCFAs is butyrate, which acts directly on the cells of the colon, reducing inflammation and decreasing the risk of cancer.

SCFAs that aren't used in the colon move to the blood, where they:

- Lower blood sugar levels
- Improve insulin sensitivity
- Promote weight loss
- Help your body absorb minerals
- Block the absorption of toxic/cancer-causing compounds

However, once a banana turns yellow, it's a sign that all of the resistant starch has been converted to sugar. That's why yellow bananas are sweeter than green bananas, and why it's better to eat your bananas when the peel is still green(ish).

If you're not a fan of eating green bananas, you can purchase green banana flour and add it to your smoothies or use it to thicken soups and sauces.

BRING BACK THE WHITE POTATO

Because of its high carbohydrate count, the white potato has been blacklisted in recent years. But while it's often shrugged off as a refined carbohydrate, the white potato is actually one of the best sources of resistant starch, a prebiotic carbohydrate that feeds the good bacteria in your gut.

When you eat white potatoes, the resistant starch gets broken down by bacteria and converted to butyrate, a short-chain fatty acid that reduces gut inflammation, provides energy to the cells in your gut lining, and helps repair weak spots that contribute to leaky gut.

Resistant starch is also unique because it doesn't have a detrimental effect on your blood sugar levels. In fact, replacing normal starches with resistant starches have been shown to help reduce blood sugar spikes after meals.

To reap the benefits of resistant starch, work white potatoes into your diet one or two times a week. Roast them, air fry them, mash them, bake them whole—the choice is yours. If you're on a low-carb diet and you want to benefit from white potatoes, you can also add raw potato starch to your soups or sauces to help thicken them. Raw potato starch is a supplemental form of resistant starch that contains 8 grams of resistant starch per tablespoon but no digestible carbohydrates. That means you get all of the gut health benefits of the specialized carbohydrate without any effect on your blood sugar.

#55

COOK AND COOL YOUR STARCHES

Some starchy foods, like rice, oatmeal, and potatoes, get even higher in resistant starch when they cool down. For example, rice that has been cooked and then cooled is higher in resistant starch than rice that's eaten as soon as it's done cooking.

To really hack these foods for gut health, cook your starches in advance, let them cool down in the refrigerator, and then eat them later—or the next day. You don't have to eat them cold, though. Once they've been cooked and then cooled, they have more resistant starch and you can reheat them any way you want.

This is even more of a reason to do some meal prep. You can make a big batch of rice or roasted potatoes on a Sunday and then pair them with some nonstarchy vegetables and a lean protein all week.

Do this for:

- Rice
- White potatoes
- Sweet potatoes
- Pasta
- Oats
- Beans

Hint: If you want to reheat potatoes, you can bring back some of their freshly cooked appeal by air frying them.

CONSIDER GOING GLUTEN-FREE

Gluten can negatively affect your gut in a number of ways:

1. Gluten changes the balance of bacteria in your gut, increasing bad bacteria while decreasing good bacteria.
2. Gluten triggers part of the immune system in your gut called the gut-associated lymphoid tissue (GALT). When this is constantly turned on, it can lead to an overactive immune response and chronic inflammation.
3. Gluten stimulates the release of antibodies that break down an enzyme called tissue transglutaminase. This enzyme keeps your intestinal lining healthy, and when it's being attacked, it leaves you vulnerable to leaky gut and nutrient deficiencies.

While the severity of the damage depends on how sensitive you are, there seems to be at least some negative effects across the board. For example, individuals who don't officially have a gluten sensitivity might only experience gas, bloating, and/or stomach cramps after eating gluten, while people who have a severe gluten intolerance or celiac disease may end up with physical gut damage and an autoimmune disease.

If you're having gut problems or chronic health issues that don't seem to have an explanation, cut gluten out of your diet for at least four weeks and see how it makes you feel. Some common sources are:

- Bread
- Baked goods
- Cereal
- Pasta
- Canned soups
- Beer

Gluten can also hide in things like condiments and spices, so make sure you read labels carefully.

#57

EAT YOUR OATS COLD

Compared to cooked oatmeal, overnight oatmeal—which is made by soaking oats in the refrigerator overnight, rather than cooking them—is higher in resistant starch, which contributes to better digestion and gut health.

Soaking the oats overnight also breaks down phytic acid, a natural compound that can be difficult to digest and blocks the absorption of certain minerals like iron, zinc, and calcium. Compared to hot oatmeal, overnight oatmeal is easier to digest and tends to cause less digestive upset in anyone sensitive to grains.

Another bonus is that you can prepare overnight oatmeal in minutes without even touching your stove, which makes breakfast meal prep simple. You can make five servings in Mason jars, close them up, put them in the refrigerator, and have a convenient to-go breakfast for the whole week.

Here's an easy gut-health boosting recipe to get you started. In a Mason jar (you can use as many as you like), mix together:

- 1/3 cup rolled oats
- 1 teaspoon chia seeds
- 3/4 cup unsweetened almond milk
- 1/2 slightly underripe medium banana, sliced
- 1 tablespoon crushed walnuts
- 1/4 teaspoon ground cinnamon
- 2 scoops vanilla protein powder

Let sit in the refrigerator at least four hours. Eat cold.

You can use your own combination of ingredients to make an overnight oatmeal that really gets your mouth watering.

WONDER AT THE POWER OF WALNUTS

A 2018 study published in the *Journal of Nutrition* found that eating walnuts daily could increase levels of three major bacteria—*Faecalibacterium*, *Roseburia*, and *Clostridium*—in your gut. Why is that good? All three of these bacteria produce a short-chain fatty acid called butyrate, which helps improve colon health. *Faecalibacterium* also acts as a probiotic, decreases inflammation, and improves insulin sensitivity. The walnuts also decreased specific bile acids, called secondary bile acids, that have been linked to the development of colon cancer.

Another study that was published in the *Journal of Nutrition* in 2020 found that eating 2 to 3 ounces of walnuts per day increased different gut bacteria. One of which, *Roseburia*, helps protect the gut lining and decrease the risk of leaky gut. Other bacteria that were increased were *Eubacterium eligens*, *Butyricicoccus*, and *Lachnospiraceae*.

Together, these bacteria have an effect on your blood pressure, total cholesterol, and non-HDL cholesterol. When they increase, your risk of heart disease goes down. Researchers went on to say that this increase in gut bacteria may be the reason, or at least part of the reason, walnuts are so good for your heart.

The participants in the study ate about twenty-eight to forty-two walnut halves daily. You can eat them straight up or blend them into smoothies. Spread walnut butter on your green(ish) bananas or drizzle it into your overnight oats.

BREAK OUT THE BRAZIL NUTS

Selenium is a mineral that doesn't get much attention, even though approximately five hundred million to one billion people worldwide are deficient. Selenium ensures that your gut has a healthy response to inflammation. A deficiency can increase the effects of stress and inflammation, damaging the gut and potentially causing leaky gut. Selenium deficiency has also been connected to a higher risk of inflammatory bowel diseases, like Crohn's disease and ulcerative colitis.

Selenium is also critical for a healthy thyroid and for converting the thyroid hormone T4 into T3. If you don't have enough selenium in your body, your thyroid doesn't work properly and you can eventually develop hypothyroidism. There are currently three million new cases per year and many more that go undiagnosed and under the radar. Doctors have discovered that many people who present with hypothyroidism or the beginning stages of thyroid disease are actually deficient in selenium, and correcting this deficiency can reverse symptoms.

But where do Brazil nuts come in? A single Brazil nut—yes, just one nut—contains almost double the entire amount of selenium that you need for the entire day. Adults need 55 micrograms of selenium each day, and one Brazil nut has 68 to 91 micrograms, depending on where and how it's grown.

#60

PRIORITIZE PLENTY OF FATS

In the 1990s, dietary fat was blackballed. Nutrition and health experts said it was bad for you and that consuming it was the main reason people got fat, so everyone started avoiding it. Several years later, after an increase in unhealthy, constipated people, the experts started to change their tune. As such, we now know that fat isn't as bad as was once believed. In fact, it's not only "not bad," it turns out that it's actually pretty good for you.

You need fat to stay healthy. This is especially true of your nervous system and your digestive tract. Fats play a role in stimulating motility, or the movement of digestive material through your intestines. When you eat a meal that contains fat, it sends a signal from your stomach and small intestine to your colon through a nerve signal called the gastrocolic reflex. This signal turns the muscular contractions in your intestine on and starts moving things along. When you follow a low-fat diet, this signal is slower to kick in, and you might notice that your digestive system doesn't seem to move as well.

An adequate intake of healthy fats is also vital to the proper absorption of vitamin A, a fat-soluble vitamin that helps keep your epithelial cells in your intestines healthy. Your intestinal epithelial cells help absorb nutrients and maintain a healthy relationship between you and your gut bacteria.

If you feel like things are a little backed up, try adding some more healthy fats to your meals. Some good options are:

- Avocados
- Eggs
- Olives and olive oil
- Coconut and coconut oil
- Nut butters
- Fatty fish like salmon

INCREASE THOSE OMEGA-3S

When it comes to gut health, fiber gets a lot of attention, but healthy fats are just as crucial to your gut microbiome. Research shows that omega-3 fatty acids increase the number of bacteria in your gut and contribute to bacterial diversity (the number of different strains of bacteria). In addition to this general benefit, omega-3 fatty acids specifically increase certain types of bacteria called *Bacteroidetes* and *Lachnospiraceae*, which have been shown to be deficient in people with irritable bowel syndrome and inflammatory bowel diseases.

Omega-3 fatty acids also:

- Improve your cholesterol profile
- Lower blood pressure
- Decrease your risk of heart disease
- Make your bones stronger
- Alleviate symptoms of rheumatoid arthritis
- Reduce your risk of memory loss and dementia

Lots of omega-3 fatty acid supplements, like high-quality fish oil, are available over the counter, but the best way to boost your intake is through nutrient-rich foods like:

- Salmon
- Mackerel
- Herring
- Sea bass
- Sardines
- Tuna
- Flaxseeds and flaxseed oil
- Chia seeds
- Hemp seeds
- Walnuts
- Seaweed and algae

To ensure that you're getting enough omega-3 fatty acids, eat a variety of these foods at least three to four times per week.

PACK IN THE POLYPHENOLS

Polyphenols are naturally occurring plant compounds that have loads of health benefits. They act as antioxidants and have been shown to reduce the risk of heart disease, help balance blood sugar, and sharpen your brain, boosting focus and memory.

Polyphenols play huge roles in your gut health too. They have characteristics similar to prebiotics, helping prompt the growth of beneficial bacteria while simultaneously inhibiting the growth of potentially harmful bacteria or other pathogens. The bacteria in your colon also feast on polyphenols and convert them into bioactive compounds that improve health and balance your gut ecosystem.

Good sources of polyphenols are:

- Berries
- Kiwi
- Cherries
- Plums
- Apples
- Chicory
- Red cabbage
- Yellow onions
- Green tea
- Dark chocolate
- Red wine

You can help keep your gut healthy by including a variety of these foods in your diet. The more variety, the better!

CONSUME SOME CRUCIFEROUS VEGETABLES

Cruciferous vegetables are rich in fiber and compounds called glucosinolates, which are sulfur-containing substances that give vegetables like broccoli their characteristic pungent aroma. The majority of glucosinolates are metabolized in your gut. When they're broken down by gut bacteria, they release compounds that help reduce inflammation in your gut and the rest of your body.

There's also an inverse relationship between your intake of cruciferous vegetables and your risk of developing cancer. In other words, the fewer cruciferous vegetables you eat, the higher your risk of cancer becomes. Or to put a more positive spin on it, the more cruciferous vegetables you eat, the lower your risk of developing cancer. That's because glucosinolates attach to carcinogenic substances and force them out of your body through your digestive tract.

The cruciferous vegetables are:

- Broccoli
- Brussels sprouts
- Bok choy
- Cabbage
- Cauliflower
- Arugula
- Collard greens
- Mustard greens
- Kale
- Rutabagas
- Turnips
- Radishes
- Watercress
- Horseradish
- Wasabi

Try to have at least one to two servings of cruciferous vegetables per day.

#64

GARNISH WITH CILANTRO

Cilantro is more than just a way to level up your tacos. The herb also acts as a chelating agent, which is something that links to heavy metals and helps your body eliminate them. Compounds in cilantro react to heavy metal ions, turning them into stable, water-soluble substances that your body can effectively detoxify rather than storing them in your organs.

Why is this important? Heavy metals kill good bacteria, increase inflammation, and contribute to leaky gut. You're likely exposed to them more than you realize—through the food you eat, the things you put on your skin, and your environment.

But chelating agents like cilantro can protect your gut, so it's important that you include them in your diet. For example, when you combine fish like tuna or rice, which is known for containing arsenic, with cilantro, the cilantro helps negate the effect the heavy metals can have on your body.

Cilantro isn't the only chelating agent, though, so if you don't like it, or you're one of those people who tastes soap when they eat cilantro (that's a real thing), you can get similar benefits from:

- Chlorella
- Spirulina
- Curry
- Garlic
- Atlantic dulse
- Wild blueberries
- Probiotics

#65

CHOOSE YOUR FISH CAREFULLY

Mercury is a heavy metal that directly contributes to gut dysbiosis, gut inflammation, and leaky gut. But mercury is harmful in an indirect way too. The heavy metal interferes with the way your body is able to use selenium, a trace mineral.

Mercury binds to selenium and prevents it from performing its duties in your body. This can increase the physical effects of stress, contribute to gut inflammation, leave you more susceptible to leaky gut, and increase your risk of bowel disease. Selenium is also vital to brain function, so when it's bound to mercury, it can cause issues with motor performance, cognition, memory, and coordination.

When it comes to your diet, one of the biggest sources of mercury is fish. Or more specifically, large fish that eat other fish. The finger is usually pointed at big fish, like tuna. However, selenium is an often overlooked piece of the puzzle here. Selenium and mercury form a bond in your body, so if you have more selenium than mercury, the effects of mercury are minimized. And most fish, including tuna, contain more selenium than mercury. Albacore, skipjack, and yellowfin tuna have the highest selenium-to-mercury ratio.

The fish with the lowest ratio, which you should avoid as much as possible, include:

- Swordfish
- Shark
- Marlin
- Orange roughy
- Walleye pollock
- Tilefish
- Pilot whale

If you combine your fish with a chelating agent—for example, by mixing cilantro into your tuna salad—the harmful effect is minimized even further.

#66

CHEW MORE!

Digestion starts in your mouth. Actually, digestion prep begins as soon as you start thinking about food or you smell something delicious, and your mouth starts to water. That saliva is your body's way of preparing for digestion. The effort you put into chewing your food makes a huge difference in how your food is digested and how nutrients are absorbed.

Not only do your teeth physically break down food, enzymes in your saliva start to chemically break down carbohydrates and fats in your mouth. Chewing also sends signals to your brain to tell your pancreas to start releasing enzymes and digestive juices so that your small intestine is ready to do its job by the time the partially digested food gets there.

There's no magic number to how many times you should chew each bite of food—different types of food break down at different rates—but here are some general tips that you can follow:

- Chew each bite at least thirty times before swallowing.
- Chew until the food in your mouth has lost most of its texture. It should feel smooth like applesauce before you swallow.
- Finish chewing and swallowing before you take another bite of food.
- Take a few breaths in between bites.
- Don't swallow liquids with your food. Ideally, you should wait half an hour after eating to drink anything, but if you do have a beverage with your meal, keep your sips separate from your bites of food.

#67

ADD YOGURT TO YOUR DAY

Thanks to the probiotic brand Activia, yogurt is probably the most well-known dietary source of probiotics available. Yogurt is made by combining milk or cream with live, active cultures—the bacteria that serve as probiotics in your gut. Over and over again, research has shown that the probiotics in yogurt, often various *Lactobacillus* strains, help balance the gut microbiome, help you go number two, and stimulate the branch of the nervous system in your gut. The probiotics in yogurt also make it easier to digest lactose, which is why many people with lactose intolerance can tolerate yogurt without any uncomfortable digestive side effects.

Yogurt also makes a great vehicle for other gut health–boosting foods, like berries, chia seeds, hemp seeds, walnuts, and cinnamon. When you combine yogurt with these foods, you turn it into a gut health powerhouse—it contains both probiotics and prebiotics that work together to fully support your gut.

Eating a cup of yogurt per day can give your gut a boost and keep you regular. But not all yogurts are created equally. Many flavored yogurts are loaded with sugar and artificial ingredients that have the opposite effect on your gut. When choosing a yogurt, get a plain, unsweetened variety with only milk or cream and live, active cultures in the ingredient list. You can flavor it by adding your own favorite mix-ins. It's also best to choose yogurts made from the milk of grass-fed animals over those from conventional dairy farms.

COOK THOSE VEGETABLES

Raw vegetables can be tough on your gut, especially if you're low in digestive enzymes and/or stomach acid or you have irritable bowel syndrome. If you feel bloated and gassy or you experience stomach pain after eating raw vegetables, try cooking them first.

Cooking vegetables essentially starts the digestion process for you. Cooking starts to break down fiber and denature proteins, which makes the vegetables easier on your stomach and helps you absorb nutrients better. Aside from that, cooking also kills many (though not all) potentially harmful bacteria or other microbes on the food, so you have less of a chance of getting sick. Cooked vegetables like asparagus, mushrooms, spinach, and carrots are actually better for you than raw, as cooking activates nutrients and allows your body to absorb them better.

However, it's important to follow some guidelines when cooking vegetables, since heat and exposure to water can make foods less nutrient-dense. The best ways to cook vegetables are:

- Steam
- Roast
- Lightly sauté

Try not to:

- Boil
- Fry

The goal is to lightly cook your vegetables until they're tender, but not mushy. Heat, light, and water can decrease water-soluble nutrients like vitamin C and the B vitamins, which is something you want to avoid.

#69

SPROUT YOUR GRAINS

One of the reasons many health professionals recommend eliminating grains is because of anti-nutrients. Anti-nutrients are natural compounds within the grains that serve as the plant's protection from animals and insects. The purpose of anti-nutrients is to make anyone or anything who eats the plants feel a little sick, with the goal that they'll learn and stop eating the plant.

Anti-nutrients also bind to vitamins, minerals, and amino acids so that you can't absorb them properly, and they inhibit your own digestive enzymes, which makes it harder to break down the grains and can lead to digestive problems and gut issues down the road.

Enter sprouting. Sprouting, which is soaking grains (and seeds and nuts and beans) in water for an extended period of time—about eighteen hours—until they germinate, can reduce anti-nutrients by up to 70 percent. A reduction in anti-nutrients translates to increased nutrient content and easier digestibility, which means they won't bother your stomach as much.

There are other benefits too. Sprouting:

- Increases protein availability and fiber content
- Breaks down some allergens
- May increase enzymes and antioxidants

You can sprout grains yourself, or you can buy them already sprouted for you. NOW Foods, Lundberg, and Thrive Market are three brands that make sprouted grains like brown rice and quinoa. If you want to really up the nutrition content and the gut health–promoting properties, cook your grains in bone broth instead of water.

#70

SKIP CONVENTIONAL DAIRY

By far, the majority of protein in milk, or about 80 percent, is in the form of casein. But not all casein is the same. There are two types: A1 beta-casein and A2 beta-casein. When you drink cow's milk, or eat anything that's dairy-based, the A1 beta-casein is broken down into a compound called beta-casomorphin-7, or BCM-7.

BCM-7 has been connected to gut inflammation, digestive symptoms like smelly gas, bloating, and diarrhea, eczema, acne, and problems with thinking and memory. It's also been linked to an increased risk of type 1 diabetes in children, autoimmune diseases, and heart disease.

On the other hand, A2 casein has not been shown to cause any of these ill effects. But, unfortunately, modern cows have been bred to produce milk that contains higher amounts of A1 casein.

So what should you do if you want to eat dairy?

1. Find dairy products that come from cows bred to have two copies of the A2 gene in their DNA. Their milk contains only A2 casein and no A1.
2. Go grass-fed. Grass-fed dairy has a better ratio of omega-3 to omega-6 fatty acids.
3. Opt for full-fat. All of the micronutrients in dairy are in its fat, so don't be scared of it.
4. Make sure the dairy products are unsweetened. Sweetened yogurt is loaded with sugar and artificial ingredients.
5. Get your dairy cultured. Cultured dairy is dairy that has been fermented with bacteria or yeast, turning it into a probiotic-rich food that's good for your gut.
6. Go organic. Organic dairy is higher in omega-3s and lower in omega-6s. It is also free of antibiotics and hormones.

DITCH THE THICKENERS

Thickeners and emulsifiers are ingredients that are added to foods to make them thicker and/or smoother. They can be synthetic (manmade) or natural, but either kind can really mess with your gut.

Studies show that thickeners and emulsifiers may be connected to gut inflammation, imbalances in gut bacteria, and autoimmune responses that can lead to damaged gut walls and contribute to the breakdown of the intestinal lining. If you have a sensitive gut, they can also cause uncomfortable gastrointestinal symptoms like bloating, gas, and diarrhea.

In an animal study published in *Scientific Reports* in 2019, researchers found that the low-grade inflammation caused by thickeners also contributed to mental health problems like anxiety and depression in mice. While there's no way to make definitive statements about this in humans, it's still a pretty valid reason to avoid them.

If you want to make sure your gut is in the best shape possible, avoid any packaged foods that contain:

- Carrageenan
- Cellulose gum
- Polysorbate 80
- Xanthan gum

These are common in plant-based milks like almond milk and coconut milk, and other "healthier" alternatives, like nondairy ice creams and yogurt. Thickeners and emulsifiers are also commonly used in chocolate and lots of packaged foods and baked goods. Read labels carefully and avoid any foods that have these ingredients.

#72

COMBINE FOODS

Food combining is an Ayurvedic principle that involves eating only certain foods together. The underlying theory is that different types of foods digest at different speeds, so eating foods that travel through the digestive system at a similar rate will help reduce digestive upset. Another part of the theory is that your body uses different enzymes to digest certain macronutrients, and starches and proteins need a different pH for proper breakdown. When you eat foods that need different levels of acidity together, it can cause gut distress.

Although this concept has been used in ancient medicine for centuries, there's no scientific evidence that it works on a physiological level. However, people have provided lots of anecdotal evidence that they feel better and have better digestion when following these principles. If your gut seems to react to everything you eat, it's worth a shot.

Food combining means:

- Eating fruit only on an empty stomach
- Not combining starches and proteins
- Not combining starches with acidic foods
- Only eating one type of protein at a time
- Eating protein with vegetables
- Consuming dairy products only on an empty stomach

A real-world scenario would look like this:

- Chicken on a vegetable salad
- Brown rice and vegetable stir-fry
- Fruit on an empty stomach
- Salad before a protein-rich meal

#73

COOK WITH COCONUT OIL

Coconut oil has been getting a lot of attention—both good and bad—in recent years. But while many think it's best to steer clear of it because of its high saturated fat content, this oil is largely misunderstood.

When it comes to gut health, two major components of coconut oil are worth mentioning: the saturated fatty acids called medium-chain triglycerides (MCTs) and lauric acid. MCTs have been shown to increase bacterial diversity in the gut and help repair the gut lining, while lauric acid is naturally antibacterial, antifungal, and antimicrobial, so it helps kill potentially harmful bacteria and yeast in your gut to keep everything balanced. Lauric acid also gets converted into monolaurin, a natural antibacterial agent that kills bad bacteria, including methicillin-resistant Staphylococcus aureus (MRSA).

Studies also show that unrefined coconut oil, specifically, can increase *Lactobacillus*, *Allobaculum*, and *Bifidobacterium*—all beneficial bacteria species that help your gut.

Researchers who published a May 2016 report in *Nutrients* went so far as to say that MCT-enriched diets may help manage metabolic diseases, like type 2 diabetes, insulin resistance, nonalcoholic fatty liver disease, and heart disease (to name a few). MCTs have also been shown to help break down fat, increase calorie burn, and promote weight loss.

There's no single answer as to how much coconut oil you need daily, but 2 tablespoons seems to be the agreed-upon amount. If you don't like the taste of unrefined coconut oil in your savory dishes, you can melt it and blend it into smoothies, add it to your coffee or tea, and/or use it in place of vegetable oil in your baked goods.

DRIZZLE YOUR DISHES WITH OLIVE OIL

Olive oil is a healthy fat, which probably isn't groundbreaking news. But what you may not know is that the active components in olive oil—mainly, the fatty acid called oleic acid—helps balance the bacteria in your gut, promoting the growth of good bacteria and starving out the bad. Extra-virgin olive oil, specifically, has been connected to an increase in *Clostridium* bacteria, which produces short-chain fatty acids that help reduce inflammation and total cholesterol levels.

Another compound in olive oil, called hydroxytyrosol (HT), acts as an antioxidant that helps promote the growth of *Lactobacillus* bacteria, a species that's been connected to better bowel habits, weight loss, reduced risk of eczema and skin conditions, and boosted immunity. The polyphenols in olive oil also help inhibit the growth of bad bacteria like *E. coli* and help prevent bacterial infections in your gut.

All this is to say: If you're not adding olive oil to your foods, you should be. Using olive oil, especially extra-virgin olive oil, in cooking may not be the best course of action because of its low smoke point, but you can get what you need by:

- Drizzling olive oil on top of roasted vegetables
- Making a salad dressing of olive oil and balsamic vinegar
- Marinating your meat and vegetables in olive oil
- Stirring olive oil into soups before serving
- Drizzling olive oil on popcorn
- Experimenting with olive oil gluten-free cake (it's delicious)

#75

CHANGE WITH THE SEASONS

Back in the day, people used to eat only what was available to them naturally. That meant that if something didn't grow during a specific season, people didn't get to eat it. But nowadays, with commercial food production, biochemical food engineering, and food preservation, this is no longer the case. However, even though most foods are available all of the time, that doesn't mean you should eat them.

Eating food that's naturally available only during that specific season is an easy way to make sure you're eating a lot of different foods throughout the year. For example, if potatoes are only available in the fall and winter months and berries are only available in the summer, you'll switch your food often and have a more diverse diet that contributes to better gut diversity as well.

Food that's in season is also richer in nutrients and often tastes better since it has everything it needs to grow and thrive naturally.

As an added bonus, in-season produce is often less expensive since it's more abundant and easier to supply, which means you'll save some money eating this way. Eating seasonal foods also allows you to support your local farms, since small-scale farmers can only grow what the current environment and climate will allow.

You can find lots of comprehensive guides to seasonal produce online. If you search "seasonal produce guide," you'll get a quick reference list from the USDA.

#76

SAMPLE MORE PAPAYA

Digestive enzymes are an important part of your digestive system. They help break down the food you eat so your body can properly absorb the nutrients. For example, the digestive enzyme called pepsin, which is made by your pancreas, breaks down protein into amino acids. Amino acids then travel to your blood so your body can use them to build other proteins. Your body cannot use macronutrients like protein in their full form. They must be broken down to be useful.

Many digestive enzymes require stomach acid to become fully activated. So if you're low on stomach acid, it's likely that your digestive enzymes aren't working properly. This can leave you with bloating, gas, diarrhea, and stomach cramps after eating.

Your body makes its own digestive enzymes, but things like poor diet, uncontrolled stress, and inflammation of the pancreas can decrease the amount. That's where foods like papaya come in.

Papaya contains papain, a compound that acts just like pepsin in your body. When you eat papaya, you supply your body with a makeshift pepsin that helps you break down proteins and absorb nutrients more effectively. However, unlike pepsin, the papain from papayas doesn't need stomach acid to work. So if you're low on stomach acid, papayas can help you properly digest your food as you work to correct the problem.

If you have the signs of low digestive enzymes, eat about $1/2$ cup of fresh papaya on an empty stomach every day and see if that improves things. You can also find papaya enzymes in supplemental form, but if you eat the fruit, you also get the vitamins, minerals, antioxidants, and fiber that come along with it.

TRY INTERMITTENT FASTING

Intermittent fasting has gotten a lot of attention as a weight-loss tool, but as far as health benefits go, losing weight is only the tip of the iceberg. According to a 2019 study published in *Turkish Journal of Gastroenterology*, intermittent fasting can positively change your gut microbiota, contributing to better gut health.

The particular changes in gut bacteria brought on by intermittent fasting help convert white fat tissue to brown fat tissue. This is extremely beneficial, because white fat stores energy and contributes to obesity, while brown fat actually burns up energy for things like your metabolism and maintaining your body temperature. When white fat is converted to brown fat, you lose weight and also experience positive changes in your metabolic health.

Intermittent fasting also gives your digestion a break from constantly running and processing food and nutrients. This allows your body to delegate energy to other tasks, most notably a cleansing mechanism called autophagy. During autophagy, your body clears out old, damaged cells and proteins, which protects you from various health problems.

You can intermittent fast in lots of different ways, but one of the most common is called time-restricted feeding, where you alternate periods of eating with periods of not eating. The most popular breakdown is an eight-hour eating window and a sixteen-hour fasting window. For example, you would eat between the hours of 10 a.m. and 6 p.m., then fast from 6 p.m. to 10 a.m. every day.

If you're new to fasting, you don't have to jump right into sixteen hours of fasting. You can start with ten hours, then gradually increase the fasting time to eleven hours, then twelve hours, and so on, until you find out what works for you.

STOP SNACKING

Every time you eat, it triggers an immune response called postprandial inflammation. While this is a perfectly healthy and normal response, you don't want it to be turned on all the time. If this low-grade inflammation never shuts off, it can negatively affect your gut health and contribute to an imbalance of bacteria.

That doesn't mean that you can't snack *ever*, but you really don't want it to be a habit. And it's not a good idea to snack when you aren't hungry anyway, for other reasons like weight gain, increased cravings, and poor blood sugar balance, to name a few.

One of the best ways to avoid snacking is to make sure there aren't any snacks in the house. That way, when temptation arises, there will be nothing to snack on. Aside from that:

- Make sure your meals are balanced and contain plenty of protein and healthy fats so you're not hungry for snacks.
- Drink lots of water. Often, thirst presents as hunger. You may think you want a snack when really, you just need water.
- Make it inconvenient to snack. Instead of keeping snack foods on the counter or easily within reach, make it harder to get to them by putting them on the highest shelf or in a tote in your pantry. The more obstacles, the less likely you are to mindlessly snack.
- Distract yourself with something else. A lot of snacking happens just because you're bored. If you're starting to feel "snacky," call a friend or take your dogs for a quick walk. Often, diverting your attention is enough to stop the craving.

#79

EAT MINDFULLY

A meal should be something that you savor, not something you rush through while you're driving home or sitting at your desk answering emails. This is partly so you can actually enjoy your meal, but there's also a physiological reason.

Digestion is a complex process that involves a lot of hormone signaling between your gut and your brain (and the rest of your nervous system). You need to be in parasympathetic mode, also called "rest and digest," to digest your food properly. If you eat while you're still in work mode, it can cause uncomfortable symptoms like gas and bloating and make it harder for your body to absorb nutrients from the food you're eating.

Aside from that, it takes about twenty minutes after eating for your brain to register that you're full. If you rush through a meal, you may eat more than you need before your body even has a chance to tell you that it's had enough. This can lead to overeating and weight gain. It also makes it hard to eat intuitively and learn your body's proper hunger and fullness cues.

Every time you eat, put your food on a real plate and sit down at a table. If you're eating a meal at work, make it a point to leave your desk and sit down in the break room or at a bench outside somewhere. Put your phone away and turn off the TV. Fully immerse yourself in your meal instead of getting lost in distractions. Spend at least twenty minutes fully invested in your meal.

#80

SWITCH THINGS UP!

If you're like most people, you tend to eat the same things over and over again. This may be because you like how your usual food tastes, but it may also just be that it makes things a lot easier. You already know how to cook and prepare the foods you eat constantly, so there's no learning curve. That's fair enough, but aside from helping prevent food boredom, there's a reason to eat a wider variety of foods.

The food you eat not only feeds you—it also feeds the bacteria in your gut. Different types of bacteria prefer different types of foods. If you eat the same handful of foods over and over, you may be feeding only a handful of bacteria and starving the rest. This means that numbers of that handful of bacteria will grow, while the others starve and die out.

To put it simply: The more diverse your diet, the more diverse your microbiome, or gut bacteria. When you eat a variety of foods, you feed all of the bacteria in your gut and allow them to grow and multiply so you have a highly functioning ecosystem in your gut.

Different foods also have varying amounts of certain vitamins and minerals. So when you eat a wide range of foods, you have a better chance of hitting all your daily nutrient needs.

To increase food diversity in your diet, learn to cook with and eat things you usually don't. Instead of reaching for spinach and broccoli for your vegetables, try asparagus, artichoke, and Swiss chard. Swap out brown rice for lentils. The goal is to eat as many different foods in a week as possible.

Chapter 3

TAKE CARE OF YOUR BODY

Your diet is the foundation to good gut health, meaning that you can't keep your gut as healthy as it should be if you're not eating the right foods. That being said, while food is important, it's not the only solution to getting your gut in shape. Sometimes nutrient deficiencies, digestive imbalances, and/or too many bad bugs in your gut can't be addressed with food alone. In those cases, you may need a little extra support.

This chapter provides forty hacks that help you correct the most common deficiencies and imbalances that wreak havoc on your gut. You'll learn which supplements are the best for gut support and how you can choose high-quality versions rather than just grabbing a random bottle off the shelf. You'll also learn some lifestyle tips to keep your digestion regular and move your lymphatic system—a network of tissues, organs, nodes, and vessels that are intricately connected to your immune system and your gut health. While all of the hacks in this chapter are well tolerated by most people, make sure you check in with your healthcare provider before making any major changes or taking new supplements. It's also a good idea to ease in slowly, rather than trying to do everything all at once. Start by incorporating a couple of hacks and then work your way up to making all of these gut-friendly changes over the course of a few months.

MAKE THE MOST OF A MULTIVITAMIN

When discussing nutrition and gut health, a lot of focus is on macro-nutrients (proteins, carbs, and fat) and what you shouldn't be eating, but you can't have a healthy gut without making sure you're getting the micronutrients (vitamins and minerals) you need. Each micronutrient has a unique function, but as a whole, vitamins and minerals support every process in your body. And if you don't consume enough, neither your body nor your gut can function optimally.

In a perfect world, you would be able to get all of the vitamins and minerals you need from your diet. But the world isn't perfect, and nowadays, with processing and industrial agriculture, food is less nutrient-dense than ever. Even if you're drinking kale smoothies and eating your vegetables, it can be difficult to meet your nutrient needs without a little help. There's where a multivitamin comes in.

A good multivitamin provides a foundation for a healthy lifestyle. The most basic multivitamins have all of the essential vitamins and minerals that you need daily. Others include additional ingredients like herb blends, bone broth powder, and/or probiotics to help address different things like stress relief and gut health.

Some good multivitamins include:

- Designs for Health DFH Complete Multi
- Ancient Nutrition Ancient Multi
- Thorne Basic Nutrients 2/Day

Remember: The goal is to supplement a healthy diet—not take a multivitamin in place of one—so make sure you're eating healthy too.

BOLSTER YOUR VITAMIN B$_{12}$

Vitamin B$_{12}$ plays a role in balancing your gut microbiome and fighting off inflammation. But according to the Framingham Offspring Study, around 40 percent of Americans may be borderline deficient, and 9 to 16 percent are truly deficient. Vitamin B$_{12}$ deficiency is especially common among vegans and vegetarians, since most dietary B$_{12}$ comes from animal products.

If you want to keep your gut healthy, it may be helpful to take vitamin B$_{12}$ as a supplement. But since all of the B vitamins work together, it's best to take a B complex, which contains all eight of the individual B vitamins. Whichever supplement you choose, make sure it contains B$_{12}$ in the form of methylcobalamin, adenosylcobalamin, or hydroxycobalamin. These are natural forms of vitamin B$_{12}$ that are more easily absorbed and safer than other forms, according to a report published in *Integrative Medicine* in February 2017.

But there's something important to consider here too. To properly absorb vitamin B$_{12}$, you need to have enough stomach acid, intrinsic factor (a protein produced in the stomach), and pepsin, an enzyme that helps break B$_{12}$ down so you can absorb it. If your gut isn't functioning as it should, you may not be getting enough from oral supplements. In this case, you may need to see your doctor for B$_{12}$ injections.

ZERO IN ON ZINC

About one in four people—or 25 percent of the world's population—are deficient in zinc, and when it comes to your gut, that's a major problem. Zinc deficiency can directly damage your gut lining, while supplementing with zinc can restore gut lining and improve gut barrier function, essentially aiding in reversing or correcting leaky gut. Zinc also helps maintain the proper balance of bacteria in the gut and contributes to bacterial diversity. As an added bonus, zinc keeps your immune system healthy and your metabolism running as it should, so it plays a role in all areas of your health.

Your body absorbs zinc picolinate slightly better than other forms (like zinc gluconate, which is the most common form available in supplements). You should always talk to your doctor before taking a new supplement, but if you think you're not getting enough zinc—some signs are lack of appetite, excessive hair loss, diarrhea, depression/low mood, impaired memory, and white spots on your nails—you can keep your gut healthy with a high-quality supplement like:

- Thorne Zinc Picolinate
- Designs for Health Zinc Supreme
- Ancient Nutrition Zinc + Probiotics
- Pure Encapsulations Zinc 30

Dosages will vary based on your personal needs, but don't go over 40 milligrams per day. Most of these high-quality supplements contain 30 milligrams or less.

#84

ADD MORE IRON TO YOUR DIET

The bacteria in your gut need iron to grow, thrive, and multiply. So if you're deficient, that means that they're deficient too. Eventually, this can throw off your entire gut balance. Iron is also vital to the production of new red blood cells, so when you don't have enough, your body can't make what it needs, and you run the risk of becoming anemic. There are currently around three million cases of iron deficiency anemia in the US, and iron deficiency is the most common nutritional deficiency in the world.

If you're a menstruating woman, you're more susceptible to iron deficiency than men because lots of iron is lost each month during your period. That's why many multivitamins that are targeted toward women contain iron, while supplements designed for men don't. That's also why women in their childbearing years have higher iron needs than older women and men.

An easy way to make sure you're getting enough iron is to take a multivitamin that includes the mineral. If you're at risk of deficiency, or your doctor recommends that you get an additional dose of iron, you can also take a supplement. Ferrous salts, like ferrous fumarate, ferrous sulfate, and ferrous bisglycinate are the best-absorbed forms of iron. Following are listed some high-quality iron supplements (manufacturers in parentheses):

- Thorne Ferrasorb
- Designs for Health Ferrochel
- Klaire Labs Iron Chelate

#85

FIND A GOOD PROBIOTIC

Probiotic supplements contain live, active bacteria that help balance your gut and ensure the good bacteria outweigh the bad. They're an excellent tool for gut health, but it's important to take a good one. Here are some things to look for:

- **CFUs.** Colony-forming units are the live bacteria in the probiotic. Since bacteria need to be alive to help your gut, it's important. Ideally, a probiotic should contain ten million to one billion CFUs.
- **Strains.** Choose a probiotic with several different strains of bacteria. Your gut is diverse, and your probiotic should be too. You don't want to give your gut high numbers of just one or two bacteria.
- **Stability.** Heat, light, and stomach acid can all kill the bacteria in your probiotic. That's why it's important to find one that's stable. Make sure your probiotic has some type of technology that ensures it makes it from your mouth to your gut. If the bacteria are killed by your stomach acid, they don't do much good. Usually, this information will be noted right on the bottle. In addition, be sure you know how to properly store your probiotic. Some need refrigeration, while others are shelf-stable.
- **Ingredients.** When you're trying to improve your gut health, it's vital to pay attention to the ingredients in everything you're consuming. Take a look at the inactive ingredient list. Choose a supplement that contains as few added ingredients as possible.

USE DIGESTIVE ENZYMES

Digestive enzymes don't get the same amount of love and attention as probiotics, but the two go hand in hand. While probiotics add good bacteria to your gut, digestive enzymes help break down food and improve your digestion.

Your body naturally makes digestive enzymes, but if you have any of the following symptoms, it's a good sign that you may need to take some in supplemental form:

- Heartburn
- Indigestion
- Undigested food in stool
- Fatigue and/or lack of energy
- Constant feeling of fullness or a "brick" in your stomach

Digestive enzymes are also a good idea if you constantly eat on the go or you're under a lot of stress, as these actions cause your digestive system to not work as well. Typically, you'll take one or more capsules with all of your meals, but that may vary depending on which supplement you pick. Some great digestive enzyme options are:

- Designs for Health Digestzymes
- Ancient Nutrition Fermented Enzymes
- Thorne Bio-Gest
- Klaire Labs Digestive Enzymes
- Pure Encapsulations Digestive Enzymes Ultra
- Garden of Life Raw Enzymes

You can even find supplements that combine probiotics and digestive enzymes together, like the Garden of Life Ultimate Care Raw Probiotics or the Not Your Average Probiotic by Organic Olivia.

SPRAY ON THE MAGNESIUM

When it comes to supplements, the most common way to take them is by mouth—usually as a capsule or tablet—but this may not be the most effective way. Although the science isn't settled on the best way to take magnesium, there's a lot of benefit to taking it transdermally (by rubbing it on the skin).

When you put something on your skin, it bypasses your digestive system and travels directly into your bloodstream. This is a faster and more concentrated delivery than taking capsules by mouth. Research shows that taking magnesium this way can effectively increase blood levels and help correct deficiencies.

Magnesium sprays contain magnesium oil, which is made from magnesium chloride, a concentrated form of magnesium that's sourced from the ocean. Spray them on your body and they travel right through your skin and into your bloodstream, where they get to work relieving muscle tension, calming you down, and aiding in digestion. It works in the same way as nicotine or lidocaine patches, which are commonly used because of their high efficacy levels.

It's best to apply magnesium oil right after a hot bath or shower, when your pores and hair follicles are open. As an added bonus, the oil helps moisturize your skin.

DROP SOME VITAMIN D

Vitamin D is one of the hardest nutrients to get through diet. That's because so few foods naturally contain it. The richest sources are salmon, sardines, mackerel, liver, and egg yolks, and those things may not make it to your plate very often.

Studies show that more than half of Americans have vitamin D insufficiency (or low levels of vitamin D), and an estimated 82 percent of people diagnosed with irritable bowel syndrome (IBS) have low vitamin D levels. The lower those vitamin D levels are, the more severe the symptoms.

What's the connection? Vitamin D receptors throughout your colon regulate bowel inflammation. When you're deficient in vitamin D, inflammation can spiral out of control, causing the symptoms of IBS. Low vitamin D levels are also associated with colon cancer and inflammatory bowel disease.

If that wasn't enough, vitamin D is a precursor to serotonin, the neurotransmitter that helps keep you happy, and most of which is made in your gut. If your vitamin D levels are low, it can lead to depression, which may be part of the reason there's a significant connection between IBS and low mood. Vitamin D deficiency also promotes widespread inflammation, which leads to imbalances in gut bacteria, even in people who are otherwise healthy.

When choosing a vitamin D supplement, make sure it's vitamin D_3 combined with vitamin K_2. Vitamin D_3 is the storage form of the vitamin that your body can convert to the active form (calcitriol), and vitamin K is necessary to ensure that your body can effectively balance vitamin D with synergistic minerals, like calcium.

#89

THROW BACK SOME ACV

When you have chronic heartburn or GERD, one of the first things your doctor will do is put you on a proton-pump inhibitor (PPI). These medications reduce the amount of stomach acid your body produces, which is supposed to fix the problem. But unfortunately, it's not so simple.

Although it seems counterintuitive, acid reflux is often caused by too *little* stomach acid, not too much. So when you already have too little stomach acid and then take a PPI, you set yourself up for side effects like headache, nausea, diarrhea, stomach pain, fatigue, and dizziness.

If you've done an at-home test that indicates low stomach acid, your best bet for long-term correction is HCl supplementation with digestive enzymes combined with a healthy diet.

While you're working to correct your stomach acid imbalance for the long term, the short-term solution is apple cider vinegar (ACV), which can help lower the pH in your stomach (allowing you to digest food more easily) and kill off any candida overgrowth. You'll want to take 1 teaspoon in 4 ounces of water first thing in the morning and then again before each meal.

But don't take any old ACV. To be effective, it must be raw, with the "mother" intact. The "mother" is a cloudy clump of living enzymes and nutrients—and that's where all of the goodness lies. Most ACV that includes the mother will say it right on the bottle, but you can tell just by looking. ACV that's clear has been processed and won't work to correct the acid imbalance. ACV that looks murky with a bunch of stuff floating around inside is what you want.

#90

BE BITTER(S)

Digestive bitters are herbal supplements that come in dropper bottles or in spray form. They're typically made from the flowers, leaves, roots, and/or bark of naturally bitter-tasting plants like dandelion, milk thistle, burdock, wormwood, and angelica root. While they're not in mainstream use in the United States, they're a staple in Chinese medicine and commonly used to aid digestion.

Digestive bitters work by kicking on your digestion and making it easier for your body to break down food and absorb nutrients. When you put digestive bitters on your tongue, the bitter taste makes your mouth water and triggers the release of digestive fluids like stomach acid and pancreatic juices. This can help reduce bloating, gas, cramps, and nausea and make it easier for you to go to the bathroom.

Taking digestive bitters also tightens the muscle at the bottom of your esophagus called the esophageal sphincter, preventing any undigested food or stomach acid from flowing backward.

It's best to take bitters about fifteen minutes before eating. If you have drops, you can put two or three drops right into a little bit of water. If you have a bitters spray, you can spray it directly into your mouth. As their name points out, they are bitter, so your mouth will probably pucker a bit when you take them. But the more you take them, the more you'll develop a taste for them, so don't give up.

#91

BREAK DOWN BIOFILMS

Most pathogenic, or "bad," bacteria, fungi, and parasites aren't hanging out in your body by themselves. They're clumped together in a colony with other bad bugs in something called a biofilm.

To create a biofilm, microorganisms stick to a surface—like your gut lining—and then start to create a sticky, slimy film that surrounds them and acts as a protection shield. This biofilm can make bacteria resistant to antibiotics and act as a physical barrier that prevents your immune cells from discovering—and destroying—them.

Biofilms are often the reason people have recurring infections like gut infections, sinus infections, or ear infections with no other explanation. Since they're really good at hiding microorganisms, biofilms are also the reason bacteria, parasites, and fungi can go under the radar during traditional lab testing. They can also contribute to mineral deficiencies, since they use minerals like magnesium, calcium, and iron to form their sticky matrix.

If you really want a balanced gut, you need to target these biofilms. Fortunately, you can combat biofilms in natural ways by eating:

- Cruciferous vegetables (broccoli, cauliflower, Brussels sprouts, etc.)
- Oregano oil
- Garlic
- Onion
- Curcumin
- Cinnamon
- Ginger
- Cranberry

You can also take N-acetylcysteine (NAC) or a number of comprehensive supplements, like Klaire Labs InterFase Plus and Kirkman Biofilm Defense, that contain a mixture of compounds that break down pathogenic biofilms while also supporting the growth of good bacteria.

CONSIDER COLOSTRUM

Colostrum is the first fluid produced by humans, cows, and other mammals immediately following delivery of a newborn and before breast milk comes in. It develops during pregnancy and lasts for a few days after birth. Rich in protein, fat, magnesium, and vitamins like A, C, E, and B, it's often thought of as one of the most nutrient-dense "foods" out there.

Now before you scrunch your nose and completely dismiss the idea of consuming colostrum in adulthood, consider that studies show that colostrum can help repair and rebuild your gut lining, strengthen the walls of your intestines, and reverse leaky gut. That's because colostrum is also rich in antibodies and several growth factors that play major roles in muscle repair—and your intestines are muscles. Other studies show that colostrum may be beneficial for colitis (inflammation of the lining of the colon).

As far as gut health goes, colostrum has also been shown to help improve:

- Stomach problems caused by the overuse of NSAIDs
- Infectious diarrhea
- *Helicobacter pylori* (*H. pylori*) infections, which are connected to stomach ulcers

Because of this, bovine (cow) colostrum supplements have become widely available and increasingly popular. You can get them in capsule or powder form, and while your specific dosage may vary, general recommendations fall between 20 grams and 60 grams per day for gut health benefits.

#93

DO A PARASITE CLEANSE

Parasites are often thought of as a problem only in developing countries, but it's estimated that about 80 percent of Americans have parasites *right now*. Parasites can come from:

- Your pets (especially if they lick your face)
- Handling other animals
- Undercooked meats
- Raw fish (sushi)
- Unwashed produce
- Swimming in lakes
- Drinking contaminated water
- Using contaminated bathrooms

Common symptoms of parasites include:

- Stomach pain
- Bloating after meals
- Diarrhea/constipation
- Rash
- Fatigue
- Rectal itching
- Weight loss or gain
- Constant hunger
- Joint and/or muscle pain
- Anxiety
- Teeth clenching/grinding
- Chronic yeast infections

If you have some or all of these symptoms, it's possible that you have parasites.

If you suspect that you have a parasite infection, doing a structured parasite cleanse can work wonders for getting you on the path to healing. CellCore Biosciences offers two kits—a foundational protocol and a comprehensive protocol—that have everything you need to get started. You can access the protocols by registering as a customer with patient direct code 4TMNGTM0.

Of course, you should always talk to your doctor before beginning a parasite cleanse or any new supplement routine.

#94

REPAIR YOUR GUT INTEGRITY

When discussing gut health, many health practitioners refer to "the three Rs" as part of the comprehensive treatment program. These three Rs are remove, restore, and repair.

First, you have to remove things that are damaging your gut, like hidden infections or processed foods. Then you have to restore your bacterial balance by eating fermented foods and prebiotics and taking supplements. After that—an often overlooked step—is repairing your gut integrity.

With years of stress, poor diet, or bacterial overgrowth, your gut lining takes a beating and, over time, this can create holes or weak spots that are often called "leaky gut." This is a big problem because the things in your gut—or intestines—are supposed to stay there (or move out when you poop). When you have holes in your gut lining, the contents of your digestive tract can move into your bloodstream and cause a number of problems like allergies, inflammation, and even autoimmune issues.

If you overlook the step of repairing these holes and weak spots, you leave your body vulnerable and make it more likely that you'll experience recurring (chronic) problems. Certain nutrients and foods help repair your gut integrity:

- L-glutamine
- Zinc
- Quercetin
- Deglycyrrhizinated licorice (DGL)
- Aloe vera
- Marshmallow root
- Slippery elm
- Collagen

You can also find multi-ingredient supplements that are specifically designed to help repair your gut integrity.

#95

POOP EVERY DAY

If you're not pooping every day, it should be one of your top priorities to figure out a way to make that happen. Your poop is one of the main ways your body eliminates toxins, and if you're not getting it out, those toxins stay stagnant in your body instead. In addition to taking supplements like probiotics and digestive enzymes, some gentle options to get your bowels moving include:

- Drinking an 8-ounce cup of warm water with about 2 tablespoons of lemon juice (the amount you'd get from half a fresh lemon) right before bed and first thing in the morning. Rinse your mouth out after drinking it, but don't brush for at least thirty minutes to avoid damaging your tooth enamel.
- Taking a teaspoon of olive oil in the morning on an empty stomach. The oil lubricates your digestive tract and can help move things along.
- Eating a handful of prunes. Not only do prunes have a lot of fiber, but they also contain sorbitol—a sugar alcohol that has a laxative effect.
- Drinking at least twelve glasses of water per day. Constipation is more likely when you're dehydrated.

While laxatives are okay for occasional relief, you shouldn't make a habit of taking them regularly. Overuse of laxatives can lead to a condition called lazy bowel syndrome, which is just like it sounds. Your bowels start to rely on laxatives and can't function well without them, ultimately making your constipation worse.

If you do take a laxative, try a natural, gentle one that contains senna as the main ingredient.

#96

JUMP ON A TRAMPOLINE

Your lymphatic system is probably the most underrated (and under attended to) system in your body, but if you want to keep your gut healthy, that needs to change. The lymph system is responsible for isolating infection and clearing out toxins from everywhere else in your body. You have twice as much lymph fluid in your body as you do blood and twice as many lymph vessels as blood vessels. And part of your lymphatic system lives in your gut.

When your lymphatic system is clogged, the lymphatic cells in your digestive tract can't absorb nutrients and fluid properly, increasing your risk of dehydration and nutrient deficiencies. Your lymphatic system also helps regulate homeostasis of fluids and your immune system, according to a 2011 report in the *Annals of the New York Academy of Sciences*.

Unlike the circulatory system, which uses your heart to pump blood, the lymphatic system has no internal pumping system and relies almost solely on movement! If you sit all day long, as many of us do, your lymphatic system probably needs some help.

A great way to get things moving is rebounding—or jumping on a mini trampoline. Rebounding (even for just five minutes a day!) helps increase lymph flow and drain toxins from the body. According to Dave Scrivens, a certified lymphologist, rebounding has been reported to increase lymph flow by fifteen to thirty times. It's a great workout too.

And this hack is for the ladies: When you jump, wear a loose-fitting sports bra or no bra at all. A lot of lymph nodes are in the breast area, and letting your breasts naturally bounce with you is an excellent way to move toxins away from that delicate area.

#97

GET A LYMPHATIC MASSAGE

Lymphatic massages, also called manual lymphatic drainage (MLD), are a great way to manually move your lymphatic system and optimize the circulation of fluids in your body. During a lymphatic massage, the therapist pushes the lymph fluid toward your lymph nodes to help your body eliminate toxins. This also helps reduce inflammation and helps restore the balance of bacteria in your gut.

After lymphatic massages, many people experience better digestion, more regular bowel movements, less bloating, and more energy. The great thing about getting lymphatic massages is you don't have to do anything except lie there.

It's like a regular massage, but the therapist will spend more time on areas that have a high concentration of lymph nodes. Every massage therapist has his or her own technique, but usually he or she works with flat hands and applies gentle pressure in wavelike motions, pushing up toward your pelvic area or underarms (where a lot of lymph nodes are located).

The number of massages you need depends on your level of congestion and how well your body responds. Talk to a certified massage therapist to figure out the best plan for you. To keep your lymphatic system healthy in between massages, drink a lot of water, move your body regularly, and eliminate processed foods from your diet.

DON'T NEGLECT YOUR MOUTH

When you hear the word *microbiome*, you may immediately think of the bacteria in your gut, but the bacteria in your mouth are also important. Studies show that oral bacteria has a major impact on your gut health and your overall health.

For example, a 2019 study published in the *Journal of Oral Microbiology* connected periodontal disease and gingivitis to poor gut health and digestive diseases. Another study, published in *Pathogens and Disease* in 2020, connected disease-causing oral bacteria like *Porphyromonas gingivalis* to chronic inflammation and lowered immunity.

It's tempting to skip your biannual visit to the dentist, especially if you have a real fear of the dentist's chair. But regular cleanings are vital to keeping your mouth—and your gut—healthy. Dentists clean areas that you can't reach on your own and help identify potential issues before they become huge problems.

If you're really scared of going to the dentist—something that's quite common—check around your area for doctors who offer sedation dentistry. In between visits, keep up with your dental health by:

- Brushing your teeth at least twice a day
- Flossing at least twice a day
- Combining circular motions and back-and-forth strokes to make sure you're covering the entire tooth's surface
- Rinsing your mouth with water after you floss
- Brushing your tongue or using a tongue scraper to remove buildup and bacteria from the tongue's surface
- Using a soft-bristle brush that doesn't tear your gums apart
- Replacing your toothbrush every three to four months

#99

SKIP THE MOUTHWASH

Mouthwash commercials always show the happiest person in the world with the whitest teeth and the freshest breath smiling hugely for the camera. However, what these ads fail to convey is that mouthwash really isn't that good for your mouth or your gut.

Studies connect the active ingredient in many mouthwashes—called chlorhexidine—to disturbances in mouth bacteria and your saliva. Like antibiotics, these mouthwashes kill bad bacteria, but they also kill the good bacteria that belong in your mouth and keep it healthy. They can also change your saliva's pH, making it more acidic and actually contributing to tooth decay.

One of the main functions of saliva is to maintain a neutral pH in your mouth when you eat or drink different things. If your saliva is too acidic, it can no longer perform this role, which can lead to damage to your teeth, gums, and any tissues surrounding the area.

What does this have to do with your gut? Tooth decay can actually contribute to gut problems through what's called the mouth-gut axis. If your teeth and gums aren't in great shape, pathogenic bacteria can seep into your bloodstream, causing inflammation and systemic disease. That's why your oral care should be improving the health of your teeth, not contributing to decay.

Instead of using mouthwash, follow a regular brushing and flossing routine, and your mouth—and breath—should stay fresh. If you do use mouthwash, make sure it doesn't contain chlorhexidine. RiseWell makes an excellent alkalizing mouthwash that keeps the pH of your mouth neutral while freshening things up.

#100

EXERCISE MORE

It's not shocking news that exercising is good for you. When it comes to exercise, there's a lot of focus on your weight and heart health, but exercise plays a vital role in keeping your gut healthy too.

According to a 2019 review published in *Gut Microbes*, regular aerobic exercise can increase the amount of certain bacteria in your gut, which also contributes to overall gut diversity. The researchers speculated that this gut effect of exercise may be one of the reasons that exercise improves brain function and mental health.

While exercise can help regardless of your current metabolic status, the more physically fit you are, the more diverse your gut bacteria become. That's why it's important to make exercise a regular part of your routine rather than something you just do now and again.

If you're sedentary, start small by adding a half hour of exercise to your day a couple of days per week. From there, work your way up to including some type of physical movement every day. It doesn't have to be structured time at the gym—you can go swimming or play a sport outside. Just make sure you're moving your body, getting your heart pumping, and working up a sweat consistently.

#101

GET A NEW BED

You're probably thinking, "What does getting a new bed have to do with my gut?" But quality sleep and gut health are intricately connected. Poor sleep can negatively affect your gut microbiome and throw off hormones like melatonin. And one of the keys to getting a good night's sleep is making sure you're actually comfortable.

According to a study published in the *Journal of Chiropractic Medicine* in 2009, your sleep surface (what you're sleeping on) plays a huge role in your overall sleep quality, how quickly you fall asleep, and whether or not you stay asleep throughout the night. If your mattress is old, or you're just not comfortable on it, investing in a new one will do wonders for your gut and your overall health and quality of life.

There's no single answer to which mattress is the "best" one. When it comes to mattresses, they run the gamut from soft to firm and everything in between. Your best bet is to go to a mattress specialist or someone who can make sure you're choosing the right mattress for your body and sleep style. And don't forget to upgrade your pillow too. Your pillow helps keep your spine properly aligned so you can sleep through the night and wake up free of any back, neck, or shoulder pain.

Keep in mind that it takes about thirty days to adjust to a new mattress, so give yourself at least that amount of time to settle in and get used to things. After that, you should see a noticeable difference in your pain and sleep quality.

#102

AVOID ANTIBIOTICS

Antibiotics are often the first line of defense against sickness, but in today's world, they're widely overprescribed, and that's when problems develop. Although the point of taking antibiotics is to kill bad bacteria, antibiotics don't differentiate between the good and bad bugs. They travel through your digestive system and kill *all* bacteria, including the beneficial bacteria that keep your gut balanced.

This can lead to long-term health symptoms as well as more acute issues like antibiotic-associated diarrhea (ADD), something that affects more than one-third of people taking antibiotics. Antibiotic overuse is also connected to the development of antibiotic-resistant bacteria that are increasingly difficult to treat.

Sometimes antibiotics are necessary, but you should avoid taking antibiotics too often. They should only be used for bacterial infections like strep throat or urinary tract infections, not viral infections like the common cold or a flu. If you're sick and your doctor can't confirm a bacterial infection, ask if you can take any other steps to try to rectify the issue rather than using antibiotics as a first line of defense.

If you do have to take antibiotics, counteract their effect by taking probiotics with them. Don't take the two at the exact same time, since the antibiotics will kill the probiotics before they're able to get to work; a good rule is to take your probiotics at least two hours before or two hours after your antibiotics.

One great probiotic option during antibiotic use is Florastor. It contains a unique strain of bacteria called *Saccharomyces boulardii* lyo CNCM I-745 that has been shown to be effective at repopulating the gut during and after antibiotic use.

DRINK YOUR HEARTBURN RELIEF

When you have heartburn or indigestion, antacids may provide a little relief in the moment, but over time, they can do more harm than good. Antacids are made from calcium carbonate, magnesium hydroxide, aluminum hydroxide, and/or sodium bicarbonate—bases that neutralize your stomach acid. The theory is that neutralizing your stomach acid will help eliminate the burning and discomfort from heartburn, indigestion, nausea, and upset stomach. While this may work in the short term, it's not a long-term solution.

Your stomach acid is acidic for good reason. One of its functions is to help break down the food you eat, so antacids can significantly diminish your stomach's ability to do its job. This can give you a feeling like there's always a brick in your stomach, since your food is only partially digested.

Stomach acid also helps control the balance of bacteria in your gut by killing off bad bacteria and preventing them from taking over the good bacteria. Decreased stomach acid increases the risk that you'll develop an intestinal infection. According to researchers who published a study in *Gut*, antacids give pathogenic bacteria like *Clostridium difficile* more of a chance to grow.

Instead of taking an antacid next time you get heartburn or indigestion, you can try:

- Peppermint, chamomile, fennel, or ginger tea
- Warm lemon water
- A teaspoon of apple cider vinegar in water

If you have chronic heartburn, these are short-term solutions to the problem. The long-term solution is diligently working on fixing your gut health, since that's where heartburn stems from.

#104

SIP ON PEPPERMINT TEA

The next time you want a nightcap or you're dealing with after-dinner cravings, reach for some peppermint tea. Peppermint helps relax the muscles in your digestive system, which can relieve digestive symptoms like gas, bloating, pain, and indigestion. When your digestive system is relaxed, you're also able to digest food better.

Some studies that show that taking peppermint oil supplements can improve symptoms of irritable bowel syndrome, reduce abdominal pain, and alleviate indigestion. However, you should never ingest essential oils without talking to your doctor or a certified aromatherapist first.

As an added bonus, peppermint has a palate-cleansing taste that leans toward sweet, so it's a great way to stave off any nighttime sugar cravings right before you go to bed.

GET NEEDLED

If your gut is out of whack, acupuncture may be able to help. In an animal study published in *Evidence-Based Complementary and Alternative Medicine* in 2020, researchers found that acupuncture helped regulate gut flora in mice, which also improved sleep by increasing melatonin (a hormone that helps you sleep) and decreasing norepinephrine (one of the main hormones involved in arousal, or keeping you awake).

The researchers pointed out that the mice with sleep disturbances all had imbalances in their gut that were resolved with the acupuncture, but what was unclear was whether the sleep problems caused the gut imbalance, or vice versa. Those details aren't really that important, though. The takeaway message is that acupuncture may be helpful for improving your gut health and helping you sleep. Another review, published in the *Journal of Internal Medicine* in 2017, reported that acupuncture may also stimulate the vagus nerve, reduce inflammation, and trigger the parasympathetic ("rest and digest") nervous system.

Keep in mind that while there's a lot of anecdotal evidence that acupuncture can help various gut disorders like nausea, vomiting, diarrhea, and irritable bowel syndrome, most of the scientific studies have been done on animals. Because of this, there's no way to make definitive statements about how this translates to human health, but acupuncture has a number of other health benefits, and it helps relax you—so it doesn't hurt to try.

GET YOUR GLUTATHIONE UP

Glutathione is an antioxidant that's vital to every single one of your body functions. It plays a role in immunity and natural detoxification and ensures that your body is able to use vitamin B_{12} properly. Without glutathione, toxins build up in your body, and you can develop a vitamin B_{12} deficiency—two things that lead to gut imbalance and inflammation.

One of your top health priorities should be making sure your glutathione levels are always healthy. Here are some ways you can boost your glutathione levels naturally:

- Get moderate (but not too strenuous) exercise, including both aerobic exercise and strength training.
- Consume sulfur-rich foods, like grass-fed beef, wild fish, pasture-raised chicken, broccoli, Brussels sprouts, cabbage, mustard greens, kale, garlic, and onions.
- Consume selenium-rich foods, like Brazil nuts, organ meats, sardines, pasture-raised chicken, grass-fed beef, and eggs.
- Get more vitamin C (from citrus fruits, kiwifruit, berries, broccoli, cauliflower, and red bell peppers) and vitamin E (from sunflower seeds, almonds, hazelnuts, spinach, and broccoli).
- Incorporate bioactive (non-denatured) grass-fed whey protein into your diet.
- Get on a healthy sleep schedule (in bed by 10 p.m., sleep at least eight hours, and no electronics an hour before bed).
- Avoid excessive alcohol intake (or avoid it completely for a while).

In addition to these tips, consider taking a glutathione-boosting supplement.

SUPPORT YOUR LIVER

Your liver is one of your biggest detoxification organs, second only to your skin. One of the most important functions of your liver is to metabolize and filter toxins and waste products and then deposit them into bile. Bile also contains enzymes and digestive juices that help you break down fats.

Bile is made in your liver and stored in your gallbladder. During digestion, it's released into the small intestine, where it helps with food breakdown and absorption. At this time, the waste and toxins in your bile are released and removed from your body through your feces. Of course, this is the scenario in a healthy functioning body.

Unfortunately, in the modern world, the liver is often overburdened with toxins and chemicals from processed foods, polluted air and water, and pesticides. As a result, it can become stagnant and unable to perform its job properly. When this happens, your detoxification pathways suffer, and toxins can build up in your liver.

Because your liver and gut are intricately connected through what's called the liver-gut axis, this buildup of toxins can lead to intestinal inflammation, altered gene expression in the gut, imbalances in gut bacteria, gallstones, and bile duct obstruction. It can even cause insulin resistance over time.

You can help make sure your liver has the support it needs through a combination of supplements and lifestyle changes, including:

- TUDCA (tauroursodeoxycholic acid)—a bile salt that may help improve digestion and liver and kidney function
- N-acetyl cysteine (NAC)
- Liver-supporting supplements: selenium, magnesium, iodine, zinc, ginger, milk thistle, dandelion, beetroot powder

#108

BRUSH YOUR SKIN

Your skin is your body's biggest organ, and it plays a major role in detoxification. While your skin is always detoxing to some degree, you can support and help this process along. One of those is dry brushing, a technique that involves using a stiff-bristle brush to gently slough off dead skin and help improve blood circulation. Dry brushing not only enhances the way your skin looks, but it also gets your lymphatic system flowing and aids in detoxification—two things that can reduce fluid retention, reduce cellulite, and boost your immunity.

Getting your lymph system flowing and opening up detoxification pathways also helps maintain balance in your gut and allows your body to properly transport and absorb nutrients throughout your digestive system. Here's how you do it:

- Get a natural-bristle brush.
- Starting at your legs (on dry skin), brush in sweeping motions all over your body, moving in the direction of your heart.
- Do this until you complete it on your whole body.
- Shower.
- Apply a natural oil, like jojoba oil or rose hip seed oil, to help soothe and moisturize the skin.

Make sure you're also cleansing and exfoliating your body two to three times a week. Exfoliating helps remove dead skin cells so that new skin can come to the surface and your skin can effectively detox.

#109

GO GREEN

Sometimes eating right and properly taking care of your gut can feel overwhelming, but if you need an easy place to start, go with this: No matter what else you do, make it a point to eat something green every day (and no, green M&M's don't count). That means green vegetables like broccoli, Swiss chard, Brussels sprouts, artichokes, asparagus, lettuce, and green peppers, to name a few.

Green vegetables are rich in vitamins, minerals, and antioxidants that support your gut and your overall health. They're also rich in chlorophyll—a natural detoxifying compound that supports bacterial balance in the gut and keeps your digestion healthy—and fiber, which promotes regularity and prevents constipation.

Of course, green vegetables won't completely compensate for a bad diet or a lifestyle that's not in line with good gut health, but making it a point to do this one thing, especially if your diet consists of a lot of processed foods or takeout dinners, is an easy way to support your gut on a foundational level while you work toward making more lifestyle changes.

#110

SCRUB YOUR GUT

You probably scrub your body every time you take a shower, but when's the last time you scrubbed your gut? Maybe never, but you can change that with *Mimosa pudica*, a flowering plant that belongs to the legume (pea) family. The seeds, which are dried and sold in supplemental form, have been used as part of traditional medicine for centuries.

Mimosa pudica seeds are mucilaginous, which means they swell and develop a gel-like consistency when they come into contact with liquid. When you take *Mimosa pudica* supplements, the seeds form a sticky gel as they move through your digestive tract. This gel attaches to whatever it comes into contact with, including the gunk and buildup on your intestinal walls. As this substance passes through your gut, all of the gunk travels with it, until it eventually comes out through your stool.

Mimosa pudica has also been shown to kill parasites and other potentially harmful microbes in your gut like bad bacteria (*E. coli* and salmonella), viruses, and fungi (*Candida albicans*). In animal studies, *Mimosa pudica* extract reduced incidences of diarrhea and increased the production of compounds that help protect the stomach lining against ulcers. While animal studies can't be directly translated to human studies, the research is promising.

It's easiest to take *Mimosa pudica* in capsule form on an empty stomach—either twenty minutes before meals or two hours after—twice a day. But if your gut is sensitive, you can start by taking it with meals and then work your way up to taking it on an empty stomach. Two great options are made by Microbe Formulas and CellCore Biosciences.

#111

MASSAGE YOUR BOWELS

Bowel massages, also called abdominal massages, are an easy, quick way to get things moving when you're constipated. Bowel massages help:

- Improve digestion
- Remove gas
- Push waste along (helping to remove blockages)
- Get abdominal fluid moving
- Stimulate a bowel movement

The good news is you can do them right at home (you don't have to see a professional therapist), and they only take a few minutes. Here's how to do one:

1. Lie down on your back with your knees bent.
2. Put your hand on the lower right-hand corner of your lower abdomen and move up along your belly to right above your belly button. Move across the top of your belly button horizontally and then down to the lower left corner of the abdomen, in a horseshoe pattern.
3. As you move your hand, use your fingertips, knuckles, or the palm of your hand to knead your abdomen gently.
4. Repeat ten to fifteen times.

#112

TAKE YOUR WORKOUT OUTSIDE

Any exercise is beneficial, but taking your workout outside has been shown to boost self-confidence and self-worth more than exercising indoors, especially for people who struggle with mental health. A study published in *Environmental Science & Technology* in 2011 found that exercising outside can decrease anger and relieve stress and tension—while simultaneously increasing energy and feelings of rejuvenation—better than hitting the gym.

When you feel confident, relaxed, and happy with yourself, these positive emotions can boost serotonin and calm your nervous system, which translates to better digestion and a more optimally functioning gut.

The next time you want to work out on a nice day, go for a hike or run through your neighborhood instead of racking up the miles on a treadmill. Being outside in general and seeing flowers, greenery, and trees has a positive effect on the brain, even if you're not working up a sweat. If the sun is shining, you'll also get some exposure to vitamin D, which also helps balance your gut, so it's an excellent way to light two candles with one flame.

#113

GEAR UP ON GLUTAMINE

Glutamine is the most abundant amino acid in the human body, and although your entire body needs it, a whopping 30 percent of the total concentration is found in your gut. One of glutamine's primary functions is to keep the lining of the small intestine healthy and free of any damage. Being low on glutamine can increase your risk of developing leaky gut, causing a variety of symptoms, including diarrhea, constipation, bloating, gas, abdominal pain, headaches, memory loss, fatigue, and brain fog.

Although glutamine isn't discussed as often as other vitamins and minerals, it's so vital for keeping your gut healthy that researchers in a 2017 review published in the *International Journal of Molecular Sciences* described it as the most important nutrient for leaky gut syndrome.

L-glutamine and D-glutamine are the two forms of glutamine. Supplements contain L-glutamine, which is the form your body can use. While dosages differ based on your individual needs, it's best to take L-glutamine in powder form, since your body can digest and absorb it better than capsules.

#114

STIR IN PSYLLIUM HUSK

Psyllium husk is a type of soluble fiber that's made from the husks of the seeds of the *Plantago ovata* plant. It's classified as a bulk-forming laxative, because it increases the bulk of your stool, which stimulates the muscles in your intestines to move things along, and it pulls water into your stool, making it softer and easier to pass. Unlike other laxatives, though, psyllium husk isn't habit-forming, so you can take it every day without ever developing a dependency on it. Psyllium husk is also unique in that it acts as a prebiotic, feeding the bacteria that produce short-chain fatty acids (SCFAs), metabolites that reduce inflammation and protect you from chronic diseases, like type 2 diabetes and cancer.

Psyllium husk is most commonly available as a powder that you can mix into any beverage (preferably water). It is the main ingredient in Metamucil, but for optimal gut health, you're better off taking a psyllium husk supplement that doesn't contain any other added ingredients. It doesn't dissolve completely, so when taking it, you'll want to stir it into your beverage and drink it as quickly as possible. Otherwise, the beverage will thicken and it can be a struggle to get it down. As for dosage, research shows gut health benefits when taking 7 to 14 grams per day, but the greatest benefit comes from taking at least 20 grams per day with 16.9 ounces of water.

GET THINGS MOVING WITH MAGNESIUM

When it comes to your gut health, magnesium does double duty. One form of magnesium, called magnesium citrate, acts like an osmotic laxative, which means it relaxes your intestinal muscles while also pulling water into bowels to bulk up your stool and make it easier to pass. This can give you relief from constipation or help prevent it in the first place.

Another form of magnesium, called magnesium glycinate, doesn't have the laxative effect, but it does help relax your nervous system and your muscles, something that can make it easier for you to go to the bathroom when you need to. Magnesium glycinate also helps you sleep, which also helps balance your hormones and your circadian rhythm—all musts for optimal gut health.

If you're dealing with constipation and need a dose of relaxation, your best bet is magnesium citrate. If you're going to the bathroom just fine but need some tension relief, magnesium glycinate is a better choice for you.

If you're supplementing with vitamin D (and you should be if you want optimal gut health), it's important to take magnesium with it. Magnesium helps your body metabolize and use vitamin D, so if you don't take the two together, you can deplete your magnesium and end up with a magnesium deficiency—something that can contribute to anxiety and constipation.

#116

STOP EATING BY 8 P.M.

You may have heard that it's best to stop eating by 8 p.m. to help with weight loss, but when looking into whether or not this was true, researchers made an interesting discovery. In one study published in *The American Journal of Clinical Nutrition* in 2017, researchers found that participants who ate after 8 p.m. were not only more likely to gain weight, they also didn't sleep as long as participants who ate their last meal earlier in the day. They also found that eating some foods, like tomato sauce, later at night could cause heartburn, indigestion, and other digestive discomfort that negatively affects sleep quality and rouses you awake throughout the night.

If you want to optimize your sleep quality and your overnight digestion, make it a point to stop eating by 8 p.m. at the latest. It's a good idea to cut fluids off at this time too. If you drink fluids too late in the day, you'll likely have to wake up in the middle of the night to pee. Aside from the fact that it's harder to fall asleep after you wake up in the middle of the night, this sleep disruption (even though it's brief) can disrupt your circadian rhythm and leave you feeling sleepy and with sluggish bowels the next day.

#117

STRETCH YOUR GUT WITH YOGA

Yoga seems to be the answer for everything these days. That's because it is an invaluable tool for your health, including your digestion. Here's how yoga can help:

- Certain poses stretch the body and apply gentle pressure on your gut organs, helping to move food along your digestive tract and alleviate tension in the abdominal muscles.
- As you move and twist, circulation to the digestive organs increases, promoting digestion and help with peristalsis—the muscle movements that push stool through your digestive tract.
- Yoga helps flush out toxins and ensures your lymphatic system is working properly.
- The deep breathing during yoga helps alleviate tension in your abdominal muscles, which can decrease bloating.
- Yoga also helps indirectly by relaxing your body and reducing your stress levels—all things that contribute to a healthier gut.

It's best to do yoga for digestion first thing in the morning before you eat anything or two to three hours after a meal. These are the best poses for digestion:

- Cat-Cow
- Camel Pose
- Child's Pose
- Sun Salutation
- Seated Side Bend
- Seated Side Twist
- Locust Pose
- Bow Pose

START YOUR DAY WITH A SMOOTHIE

Smoothies are an excellent way to get a bunch of vitamins, minerals, and antioxidants into your diet without a lot of effort. And unlike juicing, which removes the fiber from plant foods, smoothies include all of the fiber in a pulverized form that's easier for your stomach to digest. Another benefit is that you can fully customize smoothies to your own tastes and dietary preferences, making them an easy way to incorporate a lot of gut-supporting nutrients before you start your day. Here's a gut-health boosting smoothie to get you started:

Happy Tummy Smoothie

This smoothie combines soluble fiber, resistant starch, electrolytes, healthy fats, and collagen to support regularity and a healthy intestinal lining. You will need:

- 2/3 cup wild blueberries
- 1/2 small frozen banana
- 1/2 cup almond milk
- 1/2 cup coconut water
- 1/4 cup packed fresh parsley leaves
- 1/4 small avocado, peeled and pitted
- 1 teaspoon chia seeds
- 1 teaspoon grated fresh gingerroot
- 1 scoop collagen protein powder
- 1 teaspoon lemon juice

Combine all ingredients in a blender and blend until smooth. Drink immediately.

#119

STOP OVEREATING

You know the feeling: You sit down to your favorite meal and dig right in. About halfway through, your stomach starts to fill up, and you think, "Maybe I should stop eating," but it's just *so good* so you keep going. The next thing you know, your plate is empty and you're writhing around with stomach pain, tempted to unbutton your pants to get some relief.

Eating too much (and too fast) leads to bloating and poor nutrient absorption. Over time, it can also lead to weight gain. And when you constantly overeat, it can negatively affect the way your body responds to feelings of fullness and makes it harder for you to discern when you've had enough.

Your goal should be to eat until you're about 80 percent full, not completely stuffed. Try to pay attention to the physical fullness signals your body sends you, like:

- A tightening belly
- Increased pressure in your stomach
- Sluggishness
- Discomfort
- Gas pains

Another helpful tip is to define a hunger scale from 1 to 10. One is when you feel ravenous and 10 is when you're completely stuffed. Try to stop when you're around a 7 or an 8.

Also, keep in mind that fullness is regulated by the hypothalamus in your brain. When food fills your stomach, it sends signals from your gut to your brain that says you're satisfied and you don't need to eat any more. But this doesn't happen instantaneously. It takes some time for your brain to register what's going on in your stomach. Slow down, pause between bites, and wait about five to ten minutes before going back for seconds.

#120

LISTEN TO YOUR BODY

When it comes to optimal health, there's a lot of conflicting advice out there. But two things are always true: Your body knows what it wants, and you know your body better than anyone else.

When you're starting a gut health protocol or making any changes to your routine, you'll probably have some discomfort at first. It may be mental discomfort as your brain resists change, physical discomfort as your body gets used to a new routine, or a combination of both. But if you're doing something that doesn't agree with your body—for example, you start taking a new protein powder and you're bloated all the time, or you incorporate an exercise program but you feel dizzy when you do it—scale back on intensity or dose, or just stop doing it for now.

If you're not sure how to interpret your body's signals, it's a good idea to hire a functionally trained nutritionist who can help guide you through the process and help you make adjustments that are suitable for you.

When your gut is in disarray, your tolerance for new things is usually pretty low, but as you work to heal your gut and you experience all of the physiological balance that comes with it, you'll be able to push your limits more and more. Optimal gut health isn't achieved overnight. Depending on where you are right now, it can take months to start seeing some significant results, so listen to your body, adjust as you can, and trust the process.

Chapter 4

PRIORITIZE YOUR MENTAL HEALTH

If you're stressed, so is your gut. There's no way around it. When stress hormones are released, they suppress the good bacteria in your gut and negatively affect the function of your intestines. If you want a healthy, properly functioning gut, you have to prioritize your mental health. The hacks in this chapter teach you how to get your stress levels under control, how to train your brain to foster positive emotions and worry less, and how to improve the activity of your vagus nerve, called your vagal tone.

The vagus nerve, which is one of the biggest nerves connecting your gut and brain, is a vital component to a healthy gut. It starts at your brainstem, goes down through your stomach and intestines, and connects your throat and facial muscles. It also wraps around your heart and lungs. Almost all of the nerve fibers in your gut—around 90 percent—connect to your brain through your vagus nerve. This is what's known as the enteric nervous system, or mind-gut connection. Signals travel from your gut to your brain, and vice versa.

When you're dealing with chronic stress or regularly experiencing negative emotions, those emotions can affect your gut in profound ways, causing diarrhea, constipation, bloating, and all kinds of other symptoms. Fortunately, you can do many things to improve the signaling between your brain and your gut, and the hacks in this chapter show you how.

#121

REDUCE YOUR STRESS

Stress wreaks havoc on your entire body, but your gut is especially susceptible to its effects. Chronic stress triggers an inflammatory response that can change the composition, function, and metabolic activity of the bacteria that live in your gut.

Stress is also a major contributing factor to many chronic diseases and leading causes of death, like heart disease, cancer, respiratory diseases, and suicide. And this applies to all types of stress—physical, emotional, and environmental.

While it's not realistic to think that you can get rid of stress completely—it's a normal part of life—it's important to get your stress levels under control or figure out a way to manage them. This is nonnegotiable when it comes to gut health.

There's no one-size-fits-all approach to stress relief. You have to find the right combination of things that work best for you, but here are some things you can try:

- Taking time off work and/or reducing your workload
- Yoga
- Meditation
- Journaling
- Exercise
- Prioritizing sleep and making sure you get enough
- Stress-relieving supplements and herbs (Saint-John's-wort, holy basil, kava kava, ashwagandha)
- Breathwork

#122

TRY A LITTLE LOVING-KINDNESS

Meditation doesn't just feel good in the moment; there's research that suggests that practicing regular meditation can change the neural pathways in your brain, which can reduce anxiety and make you more resilient to stress.

And since meditation helps regulate your stress response, it can also help reduce chronic inflammation caused by stress and help improve your gut barrier function. Meditation also switches your nervous system from sympathetic mode ("fight or flight") to parasympathetic ("rest and digest").

One specific type of meditation, called loving-kindness or metta meditation, may be especially helpful. A study published in *Psychological Science* in 2013 found that loving-kindness meditation could increase positive emotions, which could positively affect your vagus nerve and in turn the parasympathetic nervous system in your digestive tract.

There's no right or wrong way to meditate, so don't get caught up in thinking that you have to do it "right" or not at all. If you're new to meditation, you can get started with one of the thousands of guided meditation videos available for free on *YouTube*.

THINK HAPPY THOUGHTS

There's an intricate connection between your gut and brain. Any emotions the brain experiences affects your gastrointestinal system. Positive emotions like happiness and gratitude have positive effects on your gut, whereas emotions like anxiety, sadness, anger, and fear can increase inflammation in your gut; change your gut microbiota; cause bloating and gut sensitivity; and slow down or speed up digestion, causing things like constipation and/or diarrhea.

Because of this, it's important to think good thoughts, but if you have negative tendencies, it's not that simple. The good news is that you can train your brain to think more positively though regular practice. Loretta Breuning, PhD, founder of the Inner Mammal Institute and author of *Habits of a Happy Brain*, recommends a six-step approach:

1. Build a positivity circuit by spending one full minute each day looking around and noting everything positive. Do this for at least forty-five days.
2. Give positive feedback to others every day. Try to avoid pointing out anything negative.
3. When you notice a negative thought, stop and replace it with a positive thought.
4. Perform small acts of kindness and pay it forward.
5. Eat well, sleep well, and exercise regularly.
6. Practice gratitude and mindfulness. Even in difficult moments, you can usually find something to be grateful for. Ask yourself questions like "What am I grateful for right now?"

The more you do this, the more your brain will naturally gravitate toward positivity and away from negativity.

#124

BUILD AN IRL SOCIAL NETWORK

Social media has made it easier than ever to connect with friends, family members, and even people you don't really know. But while social media creates an illusion that you're a part of people's everyday lives, mentally and emotionally, you're more disconnected than ever.

Studies link increased social media use with loneliness, which has serious physical effects on your health. Loneliness not only contributes to inflammation, it can also decrease bacterial diversity in your gut and contribute to imbalance. In a 2019 study published in *Scientific Reports*, researchers found that people who have close physical relationships have more strains of bacteria, and higher numbers of them, than people who don't.

Rather than connecting with your friends and loved ones through likes and comments, see them in person and share hugs and laughter. Make standing weekly or monthly plans, and do your best not to cancel unless something really important comes up.

Even if you can't see your friends or family members in person, make time to talk to them on the phone or, better yet, on FaceTime or Zoom. Have personal conversations in which you share things you don't talk about on social media, especially your struggles and difficult emotions.

Limit your social media use too. It may feel like you're connecting in the moment, but it's likely increasing your FOMO (fear of missing out)—and your gut inflammation—instead. Give yourself specific time limits for checking social media and stick to them as best you can.

#125

PUT YOUR PHONE DOWN

Cell phone overuse is becoming a pervasive problem around the world. When you're on the couch scrolling through your phone, it may seem like you're relaxing, but your brain is actually firing on all cylinders, taking in new information at warp speed. All that information has a physical effect on you.

When you check your phone, your brain releases a small amount of dopamine, a neurotransmitter that makes you feel really good. But the boost in dopamine is only temporary, and as soon as it drops again, you want more, so you check your phone again (and get another dopamine rush). This neurochemical reward system can trigger compulsive behaviors. In fact, the dopamine pathway is largely connected to the development of drug addiction.

Scrolling through social media or a news app can also stress you out, further increasing cortisol levels. If you do it often enough, your cortisol stays elevated most of the time. When you're relaxing, don't lie down on the couch mindlessly scrolling through Instagram. Keep your phone in another room, far out of reach. That way, you won't be tempted to check it.

Other ways you can limit your screen time include:

- Turning off notifications (if you're worried about missing an emergency, you can set specific emergency settings on most phones)
- Putting your phone on silent and out of sight during meals
- Not checking your phone first thing in the morning
- Avoiding looking at your phone for at least an hour before bed

#126

TRUST YOUR GUT

One of the best ways to make sure your gut is functioning as it should is to listen to what it's trying to tell you. Ignoring your intuition or "gut feelings" can create anxiety and stress that ultimately impair your physical gut function.

On the other hand, research shows that when you listen to your gut and spend less time trying to talk yourself out of something that you know is right, you feel happier and more satisfied overall—and that makes your gut more comfortable and your digestion better.

Of course, sometimes it's difficult to determine what's a real gut feeling and what's your anxiety or fear speaking. The best way to listen to your gut is to check in with your intuition and any physical sensations that come from it as well as your thoughts. Any time you feel uneasy, anxious, or confused:

- Sit in a quiet spot and breathe.
- Ask what your gut is saying. If you feel confused about the message, try to decipher whether that's real confusion, or if you're just scared to acknowledge your true feelings.
- Make a choice in your mind. Once you've made that choice, does your gut tighten or relax? If it relaxes, that's a good sign it's the right choice for you. If it tightens, you may be misinterpreting the message or not fully listening to your intuition.
- You don't have to act on your gut feeling right away, but it's a good idea to make a plan to follow through when the time is right.

#127

GET YOUR HANDS DIRTY

Although a lot of focus is placed on yoga and meditation, gardening is one of the best stress relievers out there. A 2010 study published in the *Journal of Health Psychology* found that gardening helped reduce stress to a greater degree than reading a book. For the study, participants were given a stressful task to do and then instructed to either read or get outside and garden for thirty minutes. The gardening group not only experienced greater reductions in cortisol levels, but they also completely regained their positive mood afterward.

In addition to improving your mental health, getting your hands dirty has a direct positive effect on gut health. Your gut and the soil around you have around the same amount of active microorganisms. However, your gut diversity—or the different types of microorganisms that live in your gut—is about 90 percent less than in soil.

Today's modern lifestyle puts a lot of focus on washing hands, sanitizing, and staying clean, but having close contact with soil helps replenish your gut bacteria and other beneficial microorganisms and molecules. There's also evidence that having more plants (as well as different types) around your yard contributes to a healthier, balanced gut microbiome.

The short version of this is: Go outside and start gardening. You can grow vegetables or flowers—the choice is yours. As long as you're getting your hands dirty and allowing yourself to become fully engaged in the moment, you'll reap the benefits of gardening.

If you live in an urban area and don't have the space, check online for community gardening programs in your area that give you access to some green space.

LAUGH AS MUCH AS YOU CAN

Hearing the saying "Laughter is the best medicine" may elicit a major eye roll, but there's actually scientific evidence behind the cliché. Laughter stimulates your diaphragm, the major muscle below your lungs that helps you breathe. When the diaphragm moves, it also stimulates your vagus nerve, which turns on your parasympathetic nervous system (your relaxation response). And when your parasympathetic nervous system is on, your digestion works better.

Laughter also improves blood circulation, elicits a relaxation response in your muscles, boosts your immune system, and improves your mood. Just ten minutes of laughter is enough to reap all of these positive benefits. Here are some ideas to help get you laughing:

- Watch funny videos on *YouTube*.
- Find a show that makes you laugh out loud and watch an episode daily.
- Call your funniest friend or family member.
- Get together with a friend and reminisce over something funny that happened.
- Play with your pets and watch them do funny things.

It's best to trigger a genuine laugh response if you can—there's nothing quite like a deep belly laugh that gets tears streaming down your face—but if you're having trouble, you can force yourself to laugh too. You may feel silly at first, but if you don't take yourself too seriously, you'll often find that forcing a fake laugh often leads to a real laugh.

#129

ENCOURAGE YOUR GAG REFLEX

This might be the weirdest thing you read today, but making yourself gag can have profound positive effects on your gut and your brain. Here's why: Your vagus nerve is connected to the muscles in your throat, notably the pharynx. A gag, also called a pharyngeal reflex, is a muscle contraction at the back of your throat. When a foreign object touches the base of your tongue, near your tonsils, the posterior pharynx contracts as a defense mechanism to help keep you from swallowing that foreign object and choking. But something else happens too. When your pharynx contracts, it also stimulates your vagus nerve, which in turn contributes to better gut health.

Keep in mind that vagal nerve stimulation is just like any other exercise. You can't do it once and expect to see immediate results. You have to commit to the process and follow through for several weeks before you'll start noticing some positive changes, so don't give up.

You can purchase a box of tongue depressors for this task or simply use your toothbrush when you're brushing your teeth twice a day.

#130

PUT YOUR PHONE TO GOOD USE

The average American spends just over five hours using the cell phone. That number is higher for teenagers, who often push seven hours. And much of that time is mindlessly scrolling through social media apps like Instagram and TikTok that can be major time wasters at best and serious dampers on your mental health, at worst.

It's ideal to limit your screen time as much as possible, but another option is to optimize the time you do spend on your phone by utilizing mental health apps that offer everything from guided meditations to deep breathing exercises to distraction games to cognitive behavioral therapy (CBT) from licensed therapists. One review published in the *Journal of Medical Internet Research* in 2017 looked at twenty-seven different studies on how mobile apps could affect your mental health and found that they can significantly improve the symptoms of anxiety and depression—two issues that can significantly affect your gut health.

Some of the most popular (and highest-rated) apps include:

- What's Up?
- MoodKit
- MindShift
- Talkspace
- Headspace
- Calm
- Ten Percent Happier

While there's still no substitute for one-on-one time with a licensed therapist (whether that's in person or virtually), these apps can serve to complement your self-care routine and provide you with a tool that you can use when you're at home and you're scrolling through your phone anyway.

#131

HUM ALONG

Your vagus nerve passes through your vocal cords, so when you do anything that activates the vocal cords, like talking or singing, your vagus is stimulated to some degree. However, humming is especially helpful since it sends strong vibrations through your throat and your vocal cords. Humming also requires you to control your breath, slowing down your inhalations and extending exhalations, which also stimulates your vagus nerve—a double whammy for your gut.

There aren't any strict rules about how to do this, but humming whenever you can makes a difference. You can do it while you're cleaning, making dinner, driving, and/or showering. Some sounds that are especially helpful are:

- Mmm
- Ahh
- Ooh

Instead of humming, you can also get the same effect from chanting or repeating a mantra like "Ommmm." The point is to make any kind of sound that would get your throat vibrating to stimulate the vagus nerve.

#132

USE YOUR BELLY!

Deep breathing, also called diaphragmatic breathing or belly breathing, means engaging your stomach, abdominal muscles, and diaphragm in every breath. When your diaphragm moves, it stimulates your vagus nerve, which then triggers your parasympathetic nervous system, or relaxation response. This process is officially called respiratory vagus nerve stimulation.

But because of things like stress, chronic tension, and even poor posture, most people nowadays do a lot of shallow breathing and have poor diaphragm movement. You may not give your breathing a second thought, but making it a point to breathe deeply, or practice diaphragmatic breathing, can change your life and improve your gut health.

Here's how to do it:

1. Breathe in through your nose while counting to four. While you're breathing in, picture your belly filling up with air and let it physically expand.
2. Breathe out through your mouth with pursed lips (like you're blowing out a candle) while counting to eight. Your exhalations should be longer than your inhalations.
3. Repeat ten times.

The goal is to fully fill, and then fully empty, your lungs with each inhale and exhale. One of the great things about deep breathing is that you can do it any time, anywhere, without calling any attention to yourself. If you find yourself in a stressful situation or you start to feel anxiety creeping in, focus on your breath and you will significantly calm yourself down within two minutes.

#133

TAKE A COLD SHOWER

Unless it's the middle of summer (and even then, really), you probably like to shower in warm to hot water. While that's certainly soothing and calming, research shows that acute cold exposure activates the neurons that stimulate the vagus nerve and help improve vagal tone over time, switching your body from a sympathetic nervous system state to a parasympathetic, or resting, state and helping you deal with outside stressors in a healthier way.

When you first feel the cold water on your skin, your fight-or-flight response will kick in. Your heart rate may increase and you tense up, but as you let your body acclimate to the colder temperature, this sympathetic activity starts to decline and your parasympathetic nervous system—or rest and digest response—kicks in.

As you repeatedly expose yourself to the cold water, you'll notice that it takes longer for your fight-or-flight response to kick in until, eventually, you stay pretty relaxed throughout the whole process. This adaptation response also helps the way you react to other outside stressors, like a busy work schedule or getting stuck in traffic. Instead of letting these things throw you for a loop, you learn to handle them with ease and a "brush your shoulders off" attitude—something that translates to better gut health because when you're relaxed, so is your gut.

The good news is you don't have to take a fully cold shower. Instead, at the end of your shower, when you're done with all of your washing, turn the temperature to cold for thirty to sixty seconds. It's difficult at first, but once you see how good you feel, you'll never go back.

#134

START SINGLE-TASKING

When your to-do list is really long, it's easy to get caught up in everything you have to complete. But instead of focusing on everything you have to do each day or week or month, focus on one thing—the most pressing thing—and get that done before moving on to, or thinking about, the next thing.

This is called "single-tasking" and is the opposite of multitasking. Research shows single-tasking decreases stress levels and actually increases productivity. When you single-task, you're fully engrossed in the task at hand. On the other hand, when you constantly switch tasks, it slows you down, so you usually end up getting less done and your work quality suffers. Research also shows that people who single-task actually enjoy their work more and feel less overwhelmed.

So, how do you do it? All you have to do is focus on one thing at a time and get it done from start to finish before moving on to the next task, whether that's cleaning the bathroom, completing an assignment for work, or doing your taxes. Here are some tips to help you:

- Leave your phone in the other room or on silent mode, and don't check it while you're doing your task.
- Turn off email notifications or anything that can pull you out of your flow.
- Set a timer for twenty-five minutes and work nonstop on that task for the entire time. When the timer goes off, you can take a five-minute break, but use it to go outside, stretch, or get a drink of water. Don't start another task or look at any electronic screens.

#135

SOAK IN SOME SALTS

Soaking in an Epsom salt bath isn't just a luxury, it's a necessity for your nervous system and your gut. Epsom salt contains magnesium, which soaks through your skin and gets into your blood, relaxing you on a physical level. Epsom salt also releases digestive hormones and neurotransmitters that contribute to healthy digestion and balanced mood.

In addition to helping boost your mental health and your resilience to stress, soaking in Epsom salt may help alleviate constipation. The magnesium that's absorbed through your skin relaxes your gut muscles and softens your stool, helping you go to the bathroom a little easier.

Check your Epsom salt labels, though. While added lavender or tea tree oil may smell nice, many scented Epsom salts contain synthetic fragrances that contain hormone disruptors and other gut-unfriendly ingredients. Use a plain Epsom salt or one that's only scented with real essential oils.

Take an Epsom salt bath at least once per week, but two to three times per week is better. Soak for at least fifteen minutes each time, and make sure the water isn't too hot.

#136

SING!

Your vagus nerve is directly connected to your vocal cords. Singing creates movement and vibrations that stimulate your vagus nerve and ultimately improve your vagal tone. One of the great things about singing is the types of sound waves and vibrations vary, depending on what you're singing. And when you sing really loudly, those vibrations get even stronger and have an even more significant effect.

Singing, and just listening to music in general, has also been shown to calm down the nervous system and reduce levels of the stress hormone cortisol. In a 2017 study published in *Frontiers in Psychology*, researchers measured cortisol and cortisone levels in saliva before and after singing. They found that levels immediately decreased after singing. But the catch is that the singing has to be performed in low-stress situations, so stick to shower performances rather than public concerts.

Singing also releases oxytocin, the same feel-good hormone that's released when you hug someone, especially when you sing in a group. That doesn't mean that you have to join a choir, but next time you're in the car with friends or making dinner with your significant other, turn on the radio and sing along to your favorite songs—or make up your own tunes and see what you come up with.

Even when you're by yourself, sing as much as you can. You don't need a reason, and you don't have to feel happy at first. In fact, if you're feeling stressed, overwhelmed, and/or sad, just force yourself to start singing and see how it changes your mood.

#137

LISTEN TO BINAURAL BEATS

Binaural beats are sound frequencies that can only be heard when you listen to certain sound waves with both ears. It's a little bit confusing, but here's a simple explanation:

Say you're listening to a sound frequency of 141 hertz (Hz) in one ear and a sound frequency of 130 Hz in the other ear. As you listen to the sounds, your brain syncs the difference and creates its own tone from the difference in sound frequencies—in this case 11 Hz. That 11 Hz sound frequency is the binaural beat.

Binaural beats are actually considered an auditory hallucination, since the beat isn't actually there. But even so, they have some serious health benefits. Binaural beats are said to calm your nervous system and trigger the same brain reaction that you get from meditation. They've been shown to:

- Reduce anxiety and increase feelings of relaxation
- Decrease stress
- Improve focus and concentration
- Boost mood
- Help with pain management

Binaural beats in video form are available free on *YouTube* (just search "binaural beats"), so you don't have to create the sound yourself. Just sit back and listen.

Put on noise-canceling headphones (if you have them) and listen to the beats for at least thirty minutes every day. Keep in mind that several different sound frequencies and waves are available, so it may take a little trial and error to find the best sounds for you.

#138

DEVELOP A MORNING ROUTINE

When high-performing people and high earners are asked for their number one tips on how they became successful, waking up early and going through a morning routine—whether that's fifteen minutes or two hours—is always at the top of the list. A morning routine has many benefits, like increased productivity levels, decreased stress, and improved self-esteem, but if you tailor your morning specifically for gut health, you'll get all of those benefits plus better digestion and a more balanced microbiome.

There's a saying that following a morning routine ensures that you control your morning, rather than having your morning control you. And here are some ways that you can gain control of your mental health and your gut:

- Drink a room-temperature glass of water as soon as you wake up.
- Take a probiotic.
- Leave your phone behind (don't even look at it until you're done with your routine). Go outside and stretch for five minutes.
- Go for a short walk if you can, even if it's just around your backyard.
- Meditate for ten minutes.
- Give yourself enough time to poop.
- Take a cold shower (or turn on the cold water for a few minutes after your warm shower).
- Make a gut-friendly smoothie with prebiotic fibers for breakfast (or your first meal if you're intermittent fasting).

#139

DO A BRAIN DUMP

If you're feeling stressed, anxious, and/or overwhelmed—emotions that can wreak havoc on your gut—a brain dump can help. It's a coping technique that frees up space in your mind by transferring overthinking from your brain to paper. Here's how to do it:

- As soon as you wake up, grab a pen and notebook. Try to avoid doing your brain dump on a computer or your phone.
- Spend ten minutes (or however long it takes) writing down every thought that comes to your mind. It can be your to-do list, your worries, random ideas—whatever comes up.
- Go about your day as usual.
- Right before you go to sleep, spend another ten minutes writing down all of your thoughts.

If you want to make it a little more organized, you can also do what's called a four-square brain dump:

- Divide your paper into four sections. At the top of each section, write these headings: Thoughts, To-Do List, Gratitude, Priorities.
- Under Thoughts, write down any random thoughts that come into your head without any judgment.
- Under To-Do List, write down everything you need to get accomplished that day (or even that week).
- Under Gratitude, write down things that you're grateful for.
- Under Priorities, write the top three to five things that are most important to complete.

There's no right or wrong way to do a brain dump. The goal is simply to get the thoughts out of your head so you can stop ruminating on them.

ESCAPE TO NATURE

If you're feeling stressed or overwhelmed, go outside and immerse yourself in nature. Go to the park or go for a walk down a trail and take some deep breaths.

According to a January 2020 report published in *Frontiers in Psychology*, spending just ten to fifty minutes in nature—or a natural space surrounded by some form of greenery—was enough to boost mood and improve focus as well as reduce blood pressure, heart rate, muscle tension, and stress hormones.

In another study, researchers found that more than two thirds of people choose a natural setting to escape to when feeling stressed. Even if you don't consider yourself an outdoorsy person, getting out into nature can help calm you down. You don't have to go camping or dig around in dirt. Just surround yourself with some greenery, take some deep breaths, and soak it in. And leave your phone behind (or at least in your pocket).

Bonus points if you can go outside in your backyard or somewhere that it's safe to walk around barefoot in the grass. This technique, called grounding, has also been shown to produce an almost immediate change in your nervous system, making you feel calmer, decreasing muscle tension, and lowering stress. Grounding can also help improve sleep and reduce pain.

#141

SMILE AT YOURSELF

When's the last time you looked at yourself in the mirror and really smiled? It probably doesn't happen often, but that's something that you should change. And fortunately, it's simple to do.

Just the act of smiling itself can help lower stress, boost your immune system, and lift your mood, but looking at yourself in the mirror while you're smiling can compound that effect. In the 1980s, a psychologist named Robert Zajonc divided participants into three groups. He had one group smile, another group smile while looking at their reflections in the mirror, and a third group look at pictures of various facial expressions.

While both smiling groups experienced improvements in mood, the group that smiled while looking at themselves in the mirror had the most significant boost. That's because when seeing a smile, even if that smile is your own, triggers mirror neurons that make you want to smile more. And smiling increases dopamine and serotonin, two neurotransmitters that are involved in happiness. Serotonin and dopamine also communicate with your gut (and your brain via your gut) and play a role in controlling gut function.

So the next time you see yourself in the mirror, look into your own eyes, smile, and say something positive, like:

- I am beautiful/handsome.
- I am confident and strong.
- I can handle whatever today brings.
- I am skilled and talented.
- I have a lot to offer to others and to myself.
- Have a good day today.

CLEAR OUT THE CLUTTER

Your environment plays a huge role in how you feel. When you're surrounded by clutter, your stress levels and the stress hormone cortisol increase, which moves blood away from the digestive tract and wreaks havoc on your stomach. It can also make you feel scatterbrained and less satisfied, making it harder to focus.

Clutter also collects dust, contributing to allergies and symptoms like sneezing, coughing, and wheezing. According to a 2016 report in *Gut*, dust mites also contribute to increased permeability of your gut (leaky gut), inflammation, and reduced gut function, especially if you're allergic.

If you're living and/or working in a cluttered space, make it a priority to clear your space out. Even if that clutter is behind closed doors or in a drawer, just knowing it's there can still have a negative effect on your mental health and your gut.

You don't have to tackle everything at once—that thought alone can be enough to overwhelm you—but make it a point to clear out a small space every day. Start with one area, like your junk drawer. Set a timer for ten minutes and get to work, clearing out all you can during that time. When the timer goes off, you can either stop or keep going for another ten minutes—the choice is yours.

You can also grab a trash bag and fill it with items you no longer need as quickly as you can. This can be old papers that need to be thrown away or clothing items that you can donate to someone in need. If you do this regularly, you'll be surprised at how quickly your space gets cleared out.

#143

CHOOSE YOUR THOUGHTS

Your gut is very sensitive to your thoughts and emotions. Has your stomach ever started to knot up and feel queasy when you're thinking about something stressful? That's a gut reaction to your thoughts. Over time, these types of thoughts can lead to chronic inflammation and even affect the ratio of good to bad bacteria in your microbiome.

It's normal to have anxious or negative thoughts in response to certain situations, but if you're having these types of thoughts all the time, it's time to take some of your control back.

You may think that your thoughts just pop out of nowhere, but you actually have a lot more control than you realize. Most thoughts are formed subconsciously, but they're still generated by your brain and the thinking patterns that you're used to. This is where choosing your thoughts comes in. It involves three major steps:

1. Recognize a negative thought.
2. Stop your negative thought.
3. Choose a positive, helpful thought.

Here's an example: Your thought may be, "I'm so overwhelmed. I don't know how I'm going to get all my work done." Recognize that thought, stop it in its tracks, and change it to: "I'm capable of doing my job. I just need to focus on one day at a time, and I will tackle my to-do list."

It may seem silly or unnatural at first, but the more you pay attention to your thoughts and put effort into changing them, the easier it will become and the better you'll feel.

#144

CHANGE YOUR WHAT-IFS

If you're an anxious person, a lot of "what-if" questions probably pop into your head all day, like:

- "What if I get fired today?"
- "What if I can't finish all of my work?"
- "What if something bad happens?"
- "What if I'm single forever?"

You get the point. While thoughts like these are normal sometimes, they can overtake you with worry if you let them. And here's the thing: On any given day, while you're focusing on all the negative or scary possibilities, it's just as likely that something really great could happen to you.

When you notice these what-if thoughts, change them to their positive counterpart as quickly as you can. That looks like this:

- "What if I get a promotion or high praise at work today?"
- "What if I get all of my work done ahead of schedule?"
- "What if something good and unexpected happens?"
- "What if I meet someone I really connect with?"

When you start transitioning your what-ifs to happy potential outcomes, you'll literally feel it in your gut. Over time, that knot in your stomach starts to loosen, you feel less cramped and bloated, and your digestion starts to work better.

#145

WORRY ON A SCHEDULE

If you're a chronic worrier, you probably spend a lot of time and energy ruminating on scary or anxious thoughts that never come to fruition. That's really no way to live.

When you consistently let your worries spiral out of control, it gets easier and easier to give in to them. But the more you tell your brain that it's only allowed to worry at certain times the more your worries will diminish in both intensity and frequency. This cognitive behavioral strategy has a surprisingly high success rate. Here's how to do it:

1. Schedule fifteen to thirty minutes of worry time every day for one week. Block it off in your calendar and make sure you can be alone during that time. Note: Don't schedule this time right before bed.
2. During your scheduled worry time, write down all of your worries, no matter how silly or insignificant they may seem.
3. When your worry time is over, go back to your regular routine. If worries start to pop into your head, tell yourself to save these thoughts for your next worry time. This will take practice, but do the best you can.
4. At the end of the week, look for any patterns in what you wrote. Are any of the items things you can control? If so, write a quick sentence or two on how you may be able to solve those problems. Are some items beyond your control? Try to put those worries aside and tell yourself that there's nothing you can do about them.
5. Repeat each week.

#146

DELEGATE

Stress manifests when your demands—physical, emotional, professional, and so on—are greater than the amount of time and/or energy that you have to give. As things build up and your to-do list gets longer, you start to feel overwhelmed. Tension tightens your stomach and can negatively affect your gut health.

The solution to this is to reduce your demands by delegating tasks to other people. In your professional life, that may mean passing off certain responsibilities to coworkers or saying no to extra work that you don't have time to complete. In your personal life, it may mean asking your children or partner for more help around the house or with chores.

If you're a type A personality or a perfectionist, it can be difficult to delegate tasks. After all, no one can accomplish them quite as well as you, right? Consider the saying, "Done is better than perfect." If delegating tasks means that they'll be off your mind and out of your hands (and actually get finished), then by all means, delegate away. You'll likely be surprised at how well other people do jobs that you thought only you could handle.

#147

SET SOME BOUNDARIES

Setting boundaries is an important thing to do for yourself and your gut. When you don't have boundaries, or people are constantly violating them, you may feel discomfort and/or resentment, which can trigger gut issues and an increased risk for gut infections. But setting boundaries can be hard work. Here are tips to get you started:

- **Identify your physical, emotional, and spiritual boundaries.** Make a firm line in the figurative sand about what you'll allow and what you won't.
- **Be assertive about your boundaries.** Communicate them to the people in your life and then enforce them. Let others know where you stand and what you'll tolerate. Be aware that you'll upset and disappoint people, but that's part of the process.
- **Start small.** If you're a people pleaser, you're not going to be able to go from zero to sixty overnight. Start with small boundaries, like letting people know you can't respond to texts after 8 p.m., and work up to bigger things.
- **Prioritize self-care.** When you properly take care of yourself, setting and implementing boundaries becomes easier because you also learn to love yourself more. Carve out specific times to do the things that bring you joy.
- **Get comfortable with being uncomfortable.** When you start setting boundaries, you'll feel a lot of discomfort. People will get upset with you and try to make you give in to their needs and wants. Hold strong in your beliefs and values.

As you work on setting—and sticking to—clear boundaries, you'll learn new things about yourself and what you will and won't tolerate.

#148

SAY NO

Learning to say no can be difficult because many of us feel obligated to say yes when someone asks for our time or energy. But if you're already stressed out or overworked, saying yes to something you don't want to do can lead to burnout, anxiety, and resentment. It will take some practice and commitment, but once you learn how to say no more often, you'll start to feel more empowered, less anxious, and have more time for yourself—all things that improve your mental health and, ultimately, your gut health.

This also applies to the food you eat. Food has become a way to connect with others socially, and when you're eating for optimal gut health, you avoid certain foods. Often, friends and family members will pressure you into eating it anyway. It's important for you to stay true to yourself here and let people know that you would prefer it if they didn't try to convince you to eat something that doesn't align with your goals.

In addition to learning how to say no to things you don't want to do, practice saying it without a lengthy explanation. Remember, no is a complete sentence, and you don't have to give any further details if you don't want to.

#149

VALIDATE YOURSELF

It's human nature to look for validation—defined as understanding and acceptance—from others. But sometimes validation doesn't come, and if you rely only on external sources to tell you that you're on the right track, you'll often end up disappointed.

Instead, make it a point to validate yourself. Self-validation is simply accepting your own thoughts, feelings, and decisions. It doesn't mean that you always have to agree or even like the way you're feeling. It just means that you accept things as they are without judgment.

Relying on external validation can lead to anxiety, depression, trouble concentrating, and feelings of guilt, while self-validation can increase self-awareness, build self-confidence, and calm down your nervous system—all things that contribute to gut health and a better functioning digestive system. Here's how to do it:

1. Acknowledge how you feel, and accept those feelings, whether they're "good" or "bad," without judgment.
2. Figure out what you need. Is it some alone time? A break from work? A healthy meal? Honor that need as best you can.
3. Don't define yourself by your feelings. Instead of saying "I am sad" or "I am anxious," say "I feel sad" or "I feel anxious." This small change is important to how your brain interprets the moment. One implies you *are* the feelings, while the other signifies that they're only temporary.

If you're having trouble with this, try to talk to yourself as you would talk to a friend. Would you tell your best friend to suck it up and get over it, or would you offer kindness and acceptance? Remember, this takes practice. Keep at it and it will get easier over time.

#150

FOCUS ON WHAT YOU CAN DO FOR OTHERS

You can do a lot of things for yourself to help improve your gut health, but sometimes, the way to feel your best is to do things for other people. While volunteer work benefits the recipient, it also:

- Boosts mood and improves depression
- Increases self-confidence
- Gives you a sense of purpose
- Counteracts the effects of stress and anxiety
- Reduces anger
- Improves physical health
- Provides much-needed social connections

And all of these things contribute to a healthier gut. If you've never volunteered before, you can find the right opportunity for you by asking yourself some questions like:

- What do I want to do?
- Who would I like to help—older adults, children, or animals?
- What skills do I have to offer?
- Which causes are important to me?

Once you have the answers to these questions, you can narrow down your options and start calling local organizations and nonprofit groups who can point you in the right direction.

You don't even have to volunteer with an organization to reap these benefits. You can work on a smaller scale by helping your family, friends, and acquaintances with things they need.

#151

FAST FROM SOCIAL MEDIA

Social media has become a mindless way to pass the time, but it's also become a source of stress. Studies show that excessive social media use can lead to feeling overwhelmed and unhappy, which can contribute to gut problems. But doing a social media "fast" can reduce stress levels and lead to a calmer mind (and, as a result, a calmer gut). Other benefits of staying off social media include:

- More time to do other things
- Better sleep
- More self-control
- Fewer distractions, so you finish tasks more quickly

If you want to be at your best, schedule regular social media breaks. Here are some tips:

- If you're using social media for hours a day, you don't have to go cold turkey and take a month off (although that would be great). Instead, schedule blocks of time for your fast, like between the hours of 6 p.m. and 8 p.m.
- Work up to longer breaks. Once you're used to staying off social media for a couple of hours every night, work up to full days without checking in.
- If you find it difficult to resist the urge to check your social media, delete the app during your fasting times.
- Expect discomfort and work through it. If you're on social media all the time, it will feel weird at first to ignore that urge, but it will be worth it.
- Get a friend on board. Going it alone can be difficult, but getting a friend or partner involved can make things easier.

#152

MAKE YOUR BED

In 2014, Admiral William McRaven gave the commencement speech (which has since gone viral) at the University of Texas in Austin. His biggest piece of advice to the graduating class was "Make your bed."

He followed up these words of wisdom by saying that making your bed in the morning gives you a small sense of pride and accomplishment that sets off a snowball effect for the rest of the day. When you complete that one small task, it makes you want to do the next thing on your to-do list, then another, until you reach the end of your day and you've checked several tasks off your list.

And while this may sound like just another cheesy commencement speech, there's a lot of truth behind his words. According to a 2020 survey by The Mattress Nerd, people who make their bed report feeling more productive and less stressed throughout the day. They also report better sleep at night. As you know by now, better sleep and less stress translates to a healthier gut.

It may be tempting to go straight to the coffeepot in the morning, but spend the few extra minutes making your bed before you do. It will be worth it!

#153

SWEAR IT OUT

No, that isn't a typo. While sweating it out is a good way to help reduce stress and improve your mental (and gut) health, so is *swearing* it out. Research shows that swearing can reduce physical pain, improve self-esteem, and help you bond with your social circle. On a physiological level, swearing can improve circulation, increase endorphins, and contribute to an overall sense of calm and well-being—all things that can benefit your gut.

So the next time you want to swear, do it. If you're feeling frustrated and you're doing all you can to keep the expletives from rolling off your tongue, go in your car or in your bedroom and let it out.

Just make sure that you're not swearing *at* anyone. When you swear at someone, it can cause them distress and negatively affect their mental health, and that's something you don't want. Keep your swears to yourself or vent them in a safe space with a loved one or close friend.

#154

SETTLE IN WITH A BOOK

Reading as a hobby has fallen in favor of scrolling social media or binge-watching your favorite shows on *Netflix*. But just thirty minutes of getting lost in a book can significantly lower stress levels and calm down your nervous system. Reading serves as a positive distraction that lets you escape the stress of daily life. It also requires you to get somewhat lost in the book—it's hard for your mind to focus on worries when you're trying to retain the information you just read. This is a form of mindfulness that can improve digestive symptoms, boost mood, and decrease anxiety.

As an added bonus, reading also enhances cognitive function and improves mental flexibility, which makes it easier for you to problem solve, make positive behavioral changes, and break negative habits, all things that can help you make the lifestyle changes necessary to improve your gut health.

One caveat: It's important to choose a book that's enjoyable for you to read—something that's lighthearted or interesting, but not something that makes the knot in your stomach tighten (like a true crime novel, for example). Romance or comedy might not be your preferred genre, but you may be surprised at how stress-free an easy-to-read book like this makes you feel.

#155

LEAVE THE ROOM AS YOU FOUND IT

Your brain thrives on order, and when you're surrounded by clutter or a mess, it can negatively affect your memory, concentration, and productivity levels. But clutter affects you physically too. Research shows that when your home environment is cluttered, you tend to have higher levels of the stress hormone cortisol. This can lead to a constant fight-or-flight response that hinders your digestion and lowers your immune response. It can even put you at a greater risk of chronic diseases, like heart disease and type 2 diabetes.

An easy way to tackle clutter before it starts is to make it a point to leave each room as you found it. That means that every time you leave a room, you take any plates, cups, papers, books, chargers (you get the point) that you brought in during the day. This doesn't apply if you're just going to the bathroom and then coming right back, but say you spent a couple of hours watching TV on the couch. You brought in a cup of tea and a plate of healthy snacks and curled up with a blanket and your laptop. When you leave the room for the night, fold up the blanket, gather your tea cup and plate, and put your laptop back where it belongs instead of saying you'll straighten up tomorrow. If you make it a point to do this every time you leave a room, you'll never get to the point where you have an overwhelming amount of clutter.

#156

TALK NICELY TO YOURSELF

Think about the last few things you said to yourself. If you're like most people, you have a tendency to engage in negative self-talk more often than you speak kindly to yourself. If that's the case, it's important to shift into positive self-talk, for your gut and your overall health. Positive self-talk has been linked to both emotional and physical health benefits like:

- Better digestion
- Reduced stress levels
- Increased happiness and less distress
- Greater life satisfaction
- Boosted immunity
- Better heart health
- Lower pain levels

If you're used to speaking negatively to yourself, it's going to take some time to cultivate a positive self-talk practice, but here are some tips that can help:

- Identify negative self-talk. As soon as you start focusing on the negative or tearing yourself down, say, "Stop!" and pivot your thinking into something positive.
- The next time you're in front of the mirror, say three things you like about your appearance. Do this every time you see your reflection. Try to pick new things as often as possible. This is called mirror work, and it's highly effective. Make sure you look into your eyes as you're giving yourself the compliments.
- Write positive affirmations like "I am beautiful" or "I am capable" on sticky notes and put them up throughout your house.

#157

CRY IT OUT

When you were young, you may have been told not to cry or to "be strong" by a well-intentioned adult. Though this person probably thought they were making you more resilient, they were actually doing you a disservice. Crying isn't just therapeutic, it actually has physical benefits too. There are three types of tears—reflex tears, continuous tears, and emotional tears. Emotional tears—the ones that come on when you're feeling sad, upset, or really happy—contain stress hormones, adrenaline, and other toxins that are released from the body when you cry. Crying also releases oxytocin, a hormone that boosts feelings of happiness and content, but is also a big driver behind proper digestion and gut health. That's why when you're all worked up and you finally let the tears out, you feel better almost instantly.

Emotional regulation and your gut health are also intricately connected. If you hold on to sadness, push it down, and try to "be strong" instead of letting it out through tears, it can wreak havoc on your gut, killing off beneficial bacteria and triggering chronic, low-grade inflammation. When you're sad, cry. If you're not used to letting your emotions out, you may need some help getting those tears to flow. In that case, you can try these tips:

- Put on a movie that's made you cry in the past (try *The Fault in Our Stars*).
- Listen to a sad song.
- Think about everything you're grateful for (crying from happiness is helpful too).
- Call a friend you can trust and share how you're feeling. Sometimes when you start talking about something, the tears flow easier.

#158

FACE YOUR FEARS

Anxiety is one of the biggest threats to your gut health. Aside from the immediate gut effects that anxiety has—like nausea and making you feel like you're going to poop your pants—chronic anxiety increases stress hormones that can cause gut inflammation and microbial imbalance. Ironically, gut inflammation and microbial imbalance can also make your existing anxiety worse.

If you're dealing with anxiety, one of your first priorities should be getting it under control. One of the most effective strategies is something called exposure therapy. Anxiety makes you want to avoid things, but when you give in to that urge, the avoidance feeds the anxiety, making it worse. Avoidance feels good in the moment—your anxiety makes you think you dodged a bullet—but the more you avoid something, the harder it becomes to face it.

The next time you're in an anxiety-provoking situation, face it head on instead of canceling it or avoiding it. Make it a goal to stay in the situation for five minutes—a manageable time period. From there, increase your exposure to ten minutes, then fifteen minutes, and so on. After doing this regularly, you'll likely notice that your anxiety has diminished and you have an easier time facing your fears. The key is to remain consistent. You won't see much of a change if you only do it once or twice.

Of course, depending on the degree of your anxiety, this is likely much easier said than done. You can try it on your own, but it's often a good idea to get a trained mental health professional involved in the process.

#159

CHILL OUT

When you're anxious or in the throes of a panic attack, it probably doesn't feel like much can help. But there's an easy trick you can use to calm yourself down almost immediately. The next time you feel anxiety coming on, grab an ice cube and hold it in your hand for as long as you can. When you reach your limit, put it in the other hand and do the same. This technique, called sensorial stimulation, helps divert your brain's attention away from the anxiety and forces it on the discomfort of the cold, which can bring your symptoms down a notch or two and help you regain composure. The cold also stimulates your vagus nerve and triggers your parasympathetic nervous system, the branch that controls your digestive system.

Instead of holding the ice in your hand, you can also put it on the back of your neck or suck on it, which has the added bonus of helping to alleviate dry mouth, which sometimes accompanies anxiety. If you don't have ice handy, you can splash ice-cold water on your face or drench a towel in cold water and hold it on the back of your neck.

#160

ASK FOR HELP

This one may not seem very "hacky," but asking for help when you need it is one of the most important things you can do for your gut health, and people often need the reminder. Feeling like you're carrying the weight of the world on your shoulders can take a major toll on your mental health and negatively affect your gut health in many ways. It's often difficult to ask for help, but it's vital.

This goes for small things—asking your kids to take out the trash or asking a coworker to finish up a project that you just don't have time for—but also for bigger things, like seeking the guidance of a mental health professional when you need an unbiased opinion or you feel like you need help beyond the tips and tricks you can apply at home. Whatever "help" looks like for you, there's no shame in reaching out to others for support. In fact, it's necessary.

Chapter 5

MAKE SOME LIFESTYLE AND ENVIRONMENTAL CHANGES

Everything in your life is connected—what you put in your mouth, what's going on in your brain and with your mental health, and the environment around you. If you want to keep your gut healthy and happy, you have to address the decisions you're making, the products you're using, and the air you're breathing. Everything that you're exposed to can have an effect on your gut health, whether that's positive or negative.

In this chapter, you will learn the lifestyle tweaks you can make to ensure that you're supporting your gut with the choices you make. You'll learn how things like your cookware and your personal care products affect your gut microbiome and your intestinal lining and the changes you can make to protect your good bacteria from harm. You'll also learn how lifestyle tweaks, like avoiding late night snacks or taking a walk in the morning, can balance your hormones and support your gut in all of the best ways. Many of these hacks are easy to incorporate with minimal effort, and others may take some getting used to, but go at your own pace. Over time, you can build up to creating a lifestyle and an environment that supports optimal gut health.

#161

BUY LOCAL

Buying local and supporting small businesses and farmers has always been a great thing to do for your community, but it's an excellent idea for your gut health too.

Your gut bacteria is closely related to the bacteria in the soil. When you buy a lot of large-scale commercial agriculture, like fruits and vegetables that you find in big-box grocery stores, you're buying food that originates far away from the bugs that naturally live around you.

Food that's grown this way is also lower in vitamins and minerals than freshly grown food. That's because processing for optimal shelf life and the use of industrial chemicals and pesticides can deplete the nutrients in the soil—and plant foods get their nutrients from the soil they're grown in.

Instead of doing your shopping at big-box stores, buy as much fresh, local produce as possible—and the closer it was grown to you, the better. Locally grown fruits and vegetables not only promote the growth of good bacteria in your gut, but they're more nutritious too. Fruits and vegetables start to lose some of their vitamins as soon as they're cut.

WATER AS SOON AS YOU WAKE UP

There's nothing like a hot, steaming fresh cup of coffee in the morning, but that shouldn't be the first thing you drink. Instead, get into a routine of drinking 16 ounces of room-temperature or warm water as soon as you wake up.

You don't have to chug it. In fact, it's better to sip it slowly and allow your body to absorb it. But as you get ready for your day or prepare your coffee, make sure you're getting those 16 ounces down.

Many people wake up dehydrated in the morning, and drinking water helps replenish the fluids that were lost overnight. Drinking water also helps flush out any toxins or metabolic by-products that were created while your body repaired itself as you slept, promoting natural detoxification and elimination and, often, triggering a morning bowel movement.

Studies also show that drinking around 16 ounces of water can increase your metabolism by as much as 30 percent, helping you burn more calories. That effect is increased even more if the water is slightly heated, so feel free to warm up your morning glass and add a squeeze of lemon if that helps get it down easier.

WARM UP YOUR WATER

In Ayurvedic medicine, it's often recommended to drink warm, rather than cold, water. The belief is that warm water hydrates, eliminates toxins, and cleanses your digestive system better than cold water, since it more closely matches the internal temperature of your body.

While there haven't been human studies done on this, animal studies show that cold water "shocks" the digestive system and can throw off bacterial balance and reduce immunity in the gut, while warm water optimizes the microbiome and keeps your gut functioning as it should. The animal studies also showed that warm water helped reduce diarrhea.

One thing to keep in mind, though, is that studies show that people are more likely to hit their water goals when the water is cool, rather than warm. So how do you reconcile the two?

You can drink warm water with some lemon in the morning right when you wake up and another warmed-up cup right before bed, but drink cool to cold water during the day to help you hit your goals. Remember, noncaffeinated tea counts toward your water intake too, so if you have trouble drinking warm water by itself or with lemon, you can put an herbal tea bag in it and sip it throughout the day.

#164

WAKE UP EARLIER

One of the best ways to improve your gut health is by regulating your circadian rhythm, and if you're a late riser, getting up earlier can help you do that. Plus, when you wake up earlier you give yourself more time to get things done, whether that's sneaking in a workout before your workday starts or having a hot cup of tea before the rest of your household gets up. That can help reduce stress levels, which also directly improves gut function.

There's no one answer to the best time to wake up, but most people should go to bed between 8 p.m. and 11 p.m. and wake up seven to nine hours later. That means if you go to bed at 11 p.m., you'd wake up between 6 a.m. and 8 a.m.

If you're not a morning person, here are some things that may help get you on an earlier schedule:

- Start by waking up fifteen minutes earlier each day. If you normally wake up at 8 a.m., you're probably not going to be able to wake up at 5 a.m. immediately, but you can start by setting your alarm for 7:45, then 7:30, and so on, to get your body used to it.
- Go to bed earlier.
- Put your alarm somewhere inconvenient, so that you have to physically get out of bed to turn it off.
- Use your extra morning time wisely. Do something productive, like reading, working out, or taking some quiet time to reflect and plan your day.

#165

STOP THE LATE-NIGHT SNACKS

Late-night snacking while you binge-watch reruns sounds like a good idea at the time, but when it's time to go to sleep, it's a decision you might regret.

While your digestive system is certainly capable of working on its own, gravity helps things along. When you're sitting upright or standing up, gravity helps pull food through your digestive system. But when your stomach is full and you lie down, you lose that effect, and your stomach's contents—undigested food and stomach acid—may actually travel backward into your esophagus. This is a big reason for acid reflux and heartburn in the middle of the night.

Aside from the fact that waking up to heartburn at 2 a.m. is super-uncomfortable, the disruptions in sleep can also throw off your circadian rhythm, negatively affecting your overall gut function as a result. Even if you don't fully awake from sleep, heartburn and indigestion can cause minor sleep disturbances that prevent you from ever reaching the deep REM sleep that's critical for optimal gut health.

The easiest way to combat this problem is to stop eating at least three hours before bed. This gives your stomach enough time to empty so that when you finally lie down to go to sleep, there won't be anything in it to flow back into your throat.

If you do eat before bed, use pillows or a backrest to prop yourself up a little bit so that you're not lying completely flat.

#166

SLEEP ON THE LEFT

You may already know that getting enough sleep is critical to your well-being, but did you know that your sleeping position may also play a role in your digestion and gut health?

Your stomach and pancreas are both on the left side of your body. When you sleep on your left side, both organs—and the digestive juices within them—sit naturally. This ensures that your digestion is working properly, even as you sleep. Gravity also plays a role in helping pull waste through your large intestine, from your ascending colon into your transverse colon and then, eventually, your descending colon. Since waste is moving throughout the night, it's more likely that you'll wake up ready to poop.

One study published in the *Journal of Clinical Gastroenterology* found that, because your stomach is on the left side of your body, lying on your left side can also help alleviate the symptoms of acid reflux.

- Upgrade your mattress to one that's designed for side sleepers.
- Get a new pillow that properly supports your neck during side sleeping.
- Put a body pillow behind your back to prevent you from rolling over in the middle of the night.
- Put a pillow between your knees to help align your spine as you sleep.
- Hug a pillow to keep your arms and shoulders aligned.

#167

SCRAPE YOUR TONGUE

Tongue scraping, officially called *jihwa prakshalana*, is a part of Ayurvedic self-care. Just like it sounds, tongue scraping involves using a specialized tool to remove particles and debris from the surface of your tongue.

As you sleep, your body processes everything you ate and were exposed to that day. During that processing and breakdown, toxins and waste products are formed, and some of them show up as a thick white or yellow coating on your tongue. Even if you're diligent about brushing your tongue with your toothbrush, it's possible that some of these toxins remain on your tongue.

One of the big benefits of tongue scraping is that it can help eliminate chronic bad breath, especially when you combine it with probiotic supplements. But a 2018 study published in *Complementary Therapies in Medicine* found that tongue scraping could also contribute to better gut health by helping improve digestion and alleviate constipation. Here's how to do it:

1. Stand in front of a mirror and stick your tongue out as far as you can.
2. Set the rounded end of a metal tongue scraper at the very back of your tongue.
3. Pull the scraper toward the tip of your tongue, gently scraping along the way.
4. Rinse or wipe the tongue scraper and repeat until your tongue is clear of any coating or debris.
5. Do this every morning and before eating or drinking anything.
6. After you tongue scrape, continue with the rest of your oral care routine.

#168

WAKE UP AND WALK

This one may be easier said than done, especially if you have to get to work early in the morning or you have kids. But if you can manage it, take a quick walk in the morning, right after you drink a big glass of water.

Your intestines are made up of muscles. When you walk, your core muscles contract and jump-start the muscles in your digestive system to fire up too. This helps expel gas and improve gut motility, as well as physically move your poop and any waste that's in your intestines.

It doesn't have to be a long walk, or even one where you exert a lot of effort—just five to ten minutes is enough. You can take a leisurely stroll with your dogs or go for a short, relaxing walk around your block. If you want to raise your heart rate a little, you can briskly walk down the street.

As an added bonus, exposing yourself to sunlight early in the morning—ideally, within an hour of waking up—also helps balance your circadian rhythm, which improves your gut health and helps you sleep better at night.

#169

GET ON A POOP SCHEDULE

You've probably heard of the merits of getting into a regular routine, and that applies to your poop too! Like anything else, your digestive system works best when on a predictable schedule.

That's why people who are really great at pooping are said to be "regular." They can count on bowel movements around the same time every day—and those bowel movements are easy to pass. That's the ultimate goal.

Fortunately, even if you're not regular, you can train your body to get on a poop schedule. This is called bowel retraining, and here's how to do it:

- Try to go at the same time every day (around twenty to forty minutes after eating is best).
- Never ignore the urge to go. While it's a good idea to train yourself to go to the bathroom at the same time every day, there will be times you have to go outside of that window, and you should always visit the restroom as soon as you feel the urge.
- Give yourself enough time to completely empty—spend around ten to fifteen minutes on the toilet, but don't strain or push. Try to let things happen naturally.
- Try to relax on the toilet. Leave your phone out of the bathroom and read a book or listen to some calming music instead.

If you have problems with constipation, you likely won't see immediate results with bowel training, but keep going and try not to get stressed out or frustrated (two emotions that can make going to the bathroom even harder). Change takes time, and if you stick to the program, you'll be happy you did.

CHECK YOUR POOP POSTURE

Before there were toilets, humans squatted to poop on the ground or into holes dug into the ground. That might seem primal compared to what you're used to now, but the truth is, the human body and digestive system hasn't evolved since then.

When you have to go to the bathroom but aren't ready to give in to the urge, the puborectalis muscle keeps your poop stored in a bend in the colon so you don't have an accident. Similar to a kink in a garden hose, this muscle pinches off your colon when you're sitting and standing. This is helpful when you're sitting and don't want to poop, but when it's time to go, it can make things more difficult.

On the other hand, a squatting position triggers the puborectalis muscle to relax, which straightens out the kink in your colon and allows poop to flow more freely out of your body with less effort on your part.

Some countries in Asia still use squatting toilets, which are built into the floor so you have to squat to use them. But you can easily turn any standard toilet into a squatting toilet with a squatting stool, like the original Squatty Potty or the TUSHY Ottoman. These stools sit on the floor in front of your toilet seat and lift your legs up to mimic a squatting position. This opens up the puborectalis muscle and helps you go. Squatting stools are great for everyone, but they can be especially helpful for anyone with pelvic floor dysfunction, which is fairly common after childbirth.

#171

MASSAGE DOWN THERE

While there are several slang terms for it, the official name for the area between your anus and vulva or scrotum is the perineum. The perineum has lots of nerves, muscles, and pressure points that can affect how well you poop.

In a 2015 study published in the *Journal of General Internal Medicine*, researchers from the UCLA Department of Medicine instructed fifty participants with functional constipation (i.e., constipation with no known underlying cause) to gently massage their perineum by pushing on the area lightly with their pointer and index finger, releasing, and then repeating several times.

After four weeks, the researchers checked in with the participants and found that the majority reported improved bowel function— meaning less constipation and more frequent bowel movements. They also reported a decrease in hemorrhoids and anal discomfort, likely due to less straining during bowel movements. Eighty-two percent of the participants also said they would continue to use this self-massage/self-acupressure technique as part of their long-term gut health plan.

If you're struggling with constipation, or you just want to keep things moving as well as they should be, give yourself a massage in this area daily. And don't feel weird about it! You have muscles all over your body, and just as massaging your back is a great way to improve your health, so is massaging your perineum.

#172

SOAK UP SOME SUNSHINE

Not many foods are naturally high in vitamin D, but the good news is that your skin can make vitamin D with exposure to the sun. Ultraviolet rays, specifically UVB, convert a natural form of cholesterol called 7-dehydrocholesterol into vitamin D_3—the active form of vitamin D. In fact, you get most of your vitamin D—50 to 90 percent—from skin exposure to the sun. The rest comes from your diet or supplements.

To maintain healthy levels of vitamin D, try to get at least ten to thirty minutes of unprotected sunlight exposure on your skin a few times per week. It's best to go outside between 10 a.m. and 3 p.m. and expose at least 40 percent of your skin to make sure you're getting enough sun to make vitamin D.

If you have darker skin or you're older (the ability to synthesize vitamin D in your skin declines with age), you may need to spend a little more time. A good rule is to base your time on how your skin reacts to sunlight. If you burn easily, spend around ten minutes in the sun, but if the sun doesn't have much of an effect on you, you can push it to thirty minutes or a little more.

#173

SAY NO TO NSAIDS

NSAIDs (nonsteroidal anti-inflammatory drugs) are anti-inflammatory medications that are often used to treat pain, inflammation, and fever. While they may shut down inflammation temporarily, they don't address what's actually causing that inflammation. In other words, they mask symptoms, but the underlying problem persists and never gets addressed.

Another problem is that regular use of NSAIDs—whether over-the-counter or prescription strength—can cause serious damage to your gut. NSAIDs block cyclooxygenase (COX) enzymes, which in turn block the production of inflammatory chemicals called prostaglandins.

This is a problem, because prostaglandins also play an important role in protecting your gut, specifically the lining of your stomach and intestines. Prostaglandins also help your blood clot properly. When you shut off prostaglandin production, your gut is more vulnerable and susceptible to injury, and the risk of uncontrolled bleeding increases.

While short-term use of NSAIDs may be necessary, it's not the best idea to rely on them long term. If you have a chronic inflammatory condition or you're constantly in pain, try to get to the root of the problem instead of relying on NSAIDs as a temporary solution.

Instead of using these, switch to natural anti-inflammatories like turmeric, which has been shown to be just as effective as some NSAIDs but without the negative side effects. You can take turmeric in supplemental form—usually marketed as curcumin, which is the active compound in turmeric. Make sure the curcumin in the supplement is also combined with black pepper. Black pepper contains piperine, which increases curcumin absorption by as much as 2,000 percent.

Of course, talk to your doctor before making any changes, especially if you take an NSAID prescription.

#174

DITCH THE ANTACIDS

Antacids are often the first line of defense against heartburn and/ or indigestion. While it makes sense to conclude that the acid reflux that causes heartburn is a result of too much stomach acid, too little stomach acid is actually a more common problem, and, in these cases, antacids make things a lot worse.

Antacids neutralize stomach acid while simultaneously blocking its production. They also inhibit the activity of pepsin, an enzyme that helps break down and digest protein. This combo not only hinders digestion, but according to an animal study published in *The Journal of Allergy and Clinical Immunology* in 2003, it may also increase your risk of developing food allergies down the line.

In addition, antacids have some gnarly long-term side effects, including chronic diarrhea, negative changes in your metabolism, kidney stones, and mental health changes. Aside from that, antacids don't get to the root of your problem. Antacids may relieve symptoms in the short term, but they essentially act as a bandage, covering up a problem without correcting it. If you're having chronic heartburn, there's a reason for it—it could be a poor diet, low stomach acid, too much stress, and so on—and you need to work toward uncovering that underlying issue to truly fix your gut health.

#175

LIMIT ALCOHOL

Red wine is often touted as a healthy choice that helps protect against heart disease. While it's true that the grapes it's made from are high in antioxidants, alcohol really does more harm than good, especially when it comes to your gut health.

Alcohol is absorbed in your upper intestine, and the bacteria that live there help you metabolize it. This is one reason that people have different reactions when they drink alcohol. If you have fewer good bacteria and a lot of bad bacteria, your body can't detoxify alcohol as well. Alcohol also kills good bacteria while encouraging the growth of harmful bacteria—something that can throw off the bacterial balance in your gut even more.

Of course, alcohol also intensifies cravings for processed, carbohydrate-heavy foods like pizza, which can contribute to gut problems. That doesn't mean that you have to avoid alcohol completely, but you can make more gut-friendly choices about how much you drink. When you do drink alcohol:

- Drink responsibly. Limit yourself to one or two drinks at a time.
- Choose red wine when possible. The resveratrol in it does have some positive effects on gut health.
- For every alcoholic drink you consume, have 4 ounces of kombucha. Kombucha is a fermented tea that's loaded with beneficial probiotics, so it can help protect your gut from the alcohol.
- Alternate each alcoholic drink with a glass of water to prevent dehydration.
- Always eat a healthy, nourishing meal before you drink alcohol. Bonus points if it contains prebiotic-rich foods like garlic, onions, leeks, asparagus, oats, apples, and/or flaxseeds.

#176

HANG OUT WITH MORE ANIMALS

If you're an animal lover, you probably don't need any more convincing to hang out with your pets—or even other people's pets—but here's a scientific reason: Studies show that people who own pets—or are regularly exposed to animals—have more bacterial diversity in their guts than people who have less contact with animals. Researchers who conducted a 2020 study published in *Frontiers in Cellular and Infection Microbiology* went on to say that this may lead to a decrease in allergic diseases like rhinitis, eczema, and asthma.

Another interesting conclusion—this one from a 2017 *Microbiome* study—is that babies who are exposed to pets in their first three to four months of life have a lower risk of developing allergic diseases and becoming overweight later in life, especially if the baby was born via C-section. This is significant, because babies born by C-section are typically missing key gut bacteria because they don't get the same exposure to their moms' bacteria as babies who are born vaginally.

The bottom line is this: If you're on the fence about getting a pet, it's a wise gut-health decision to give in. If you don't own a pet but like the idea of spending more time with animals—either because it helps improve your gut health or because it just makes you happier—see if there's a local animal shelter where you can volunteer regularly. And if you have a small baby, or are expecting one soon, don't be afraid to safely let your household pets near them.

#177

SWITCH YOUR CLEANING PRODUCTS

When it comes to your home, you may think the cleaner, the better. There's nothing better for your body and your health than bleached and sanitized surfaces, right? Eh, not so fast. While that smell of "clean" in the air may make you feel like you're doing something good for yourself, harsh cleaning products, detergents, and sanitizers can negatively affect your gut.

Researchers who published a study in the *Canadian Medical Association Journal* looked at the impact of cleaning products on the gut bacteria of almost eight hundred children. They found that when babies are exposed to disinfectants like multisurface cleaners at a young age, it messes with three strains of bacteria that are associated with weight.

As a result, the babies exposed to harsh, toxic household cleaners were more likely to be overweight at the age of three, while babies that weren't exposed to these types of cleaners—or babies in households that used eco-friendly cleaners—had lower BMIs when they got older.

Switch to eco-friendly and natural cleaners instead. You might not get that bleach smell, but your house will be just as clean, and your gut will thank you.

WASH, DON'T SANITIZE

During the COVID-19 pandemic, hand sanitizers earned their time in the spotlight. And while they certainly have their place, there is such a thing as oversanitizing. The problem is that hand sanitizers don't differentiate between good bacteria and bad bacteria. They kill every type of microbe that they come into contact with. And in the case of hand sanitizers, that's not only limited to the microbes on your skin.

An animal study published in *PLOS One* found that triclosan, which is one of the most common active ingredients in hand sanitizers (and is also registered as a pesticide by the FDA, by the way), can negatively affect the bacteria in your gut. That's because it's easily absorbed through your skin and your intestines, so when you put it on your hands, it makes its way quickly into the rest of your body.

While triclosan is most commonly found in hand sanitizers, it's also a popular ingredient in toothpastes, antibacterial soaps, and body washes. If you want to make sure your gut is the healthiest it can be, check your labels and ditch any sanitizing or personal care products that list it as an ingredient.

Many natural hand sanitizers, toothpastes, and body washes are just as effective. Take some time to find one that you like and make the switch. And when you can, wash your hands with a gentle soap and warm water to clean them, rather than using hand sanitizer.

WATCH WHAT YOU PUT ON YOUR SKIN

When it comes to your gut health, what you put on your skin is just as important as what you eat. In fact, it might even be more important, since the things you eat are filtered through your digestive system, while the things you put on your skin travel directly into your bloodstream.

Many personal care products don't need FDA approval prior to hitting the market. So companies can pretty much add whatever ingredients they want without many restrictions. And studies show that ingredients that are commonly used in personal care products can significantly disrupt the gut microbiome, even at low exposures. Exposure to these toxic chemicals has also been linked to cancer, infertility, asthma, weight gain, hormonal imbalances, and more.

When you're trying to hack your gut health, it's vital that you pay attention to what you put on your skin. Read ingredient labels and avoid anything with:

- Parabens (methylparaben, propylparaben, butylparaben, ethylparaben)
- Phthalates
- Fragrance/parfum
- Quaternium-15
- Sodium lauryl sulfate (SLS) and sodium laureth sulfate (SLES)
- Polyethylene glycol
- Ceteareth-20
- Triclosan and triclocarban
- Butylated hydroxyanisole (BHA) and butylated hydroxytoluene (BHT)
- Dibutyl phthalate (DBP)

DON'T BURN SCENTED CANDLES

Scented candles can certainly set the mood, but they make your gut—and the rest of your body—pretty unhappy. Most scented candles are made with a combination of paraffin wax (which is made from petroleum) and synthetic fragrances, a toxic combination.

What's arguably most alarming is that the FDA doesn't require companies to disclose what's in their fragrances. This is so that the company can protect itself from other manufacturers who may try to copy signature scents. But that means you could be breathing in a mishmash of harmful chemicals and not even know it.

Many fragrances contain hormone-disrupting chemicals that can wreak havoc on your gut and the rest of your body. These fragrances—and the burn-off from toxic ingredients in the candle—also contribute to indoor air pollution.

The good news is that this doesn't apply to all candles (but it does apply to some of the most popular brands). Many smaller companies and local candle makers use a combination of essential oils and natural waxes like beeswax or soy instead of synthetic chemicals. If you love your candles too much to get rid of them, switch to natural candles. They're generally a little more expensive, but they're safe, and the essential oils actually have health benefits too. For example, lavender and chamomile may help relieve stress and calm you down, while peppermint directly aids in digestion.

If you prefer to ditch candles altogether but want to replicate the ambiance of scented candles, get an aromatherapy diffuser and put it next to a Himalayan salt lamp or flickering flameless candles. You can also find a diffuser that emits a soft light that's just as relaxing as the light from candles.

#181

PURIFY YOUR AIR

According to a study published in *Environmental International* in May 2020, air pollution has a significant effect on the composition of your gut. Pollutants in the air can increase bad bacteria while also decreasing good bacteria. This can contribute to gut inflammation, which increases the risk of digestive disorders, weight gain (and obesity), and type 2 diabetes, among other health problems.

When you hear the words *air pollution*, your mind may immediately go to smoggy air outside, but according to Environmental Working Group, the air in your home is about two to five times more polluted than the air outside. In some cases, it can be as much as one hundred times more polluted.

But the good news is air purifiers can remove up to 99.97 percent of pollutants and allergens from your air, protecting your gut and helping maintain the proper bacterial balance. As an added bonus, purifying your air has also been shown to reduce allergy and asthma symptoms and even improve heart health.

The best air purifiers combine a HEPA filter with activated carbon filters. The HEPA filter captures bigger particles like dust and pollen, while the activated carbon traps gases like volatile organic compounds and radon.

#182

FILTER YOUR WATER

If you get your water from your town's water supply, it may be time to invest in a water filter. Many towns add chlorine to tap water in a process called chlorination. The chlorine is supposed to kill any bacteria, viruses, and parasites in the water—and it does—but when you drink it, it also kills any good bacteria in your gut.

If you drink tap water, it's a good idea to get a water filter that removes chlorine from your drinking water. A whole-house filter installs directly at your home's water supply. One of the biggest benefits to going this route is that these types of filters clean all of the water in the house, including bathwater and sink water, not just your drinking water. Even if you're drinking only filtered water, chlorine can still get into your system and mess up your gut through your skin when you take a shower or relax in a nice hot bath.

Whole-house filters can be expensive, so if you don't have the budget or you don't own your own home, try cheaper options made for drinking water. The Berkey Water Filter is one of the best countertop water filters you can buy. In addition to filtering chlorine in tap water to undetectable levels, it also filters out pesticides, medications, heavy metals, BPA, and other harmful elements without removing any beneficial minerals like calcium, magnesium, and/or potassium.

#183

SAY GOODBYE TO PLASTIC

By now, most health experts agree that plastics that contain bisphenol-A (BPA) aren't good for you. Among other negative health effects, research shows that BPA can decrease beneficial bacteria in your gut and throw off the balance of your gut microbiome, leaving you more susceptible to develop health problems like heart disease, liver disease, thyroid disease, obesity, reproductive problems, type 2 diabetes, and reduced immune function. What's more, this negative effect can be passed down through generations, meaning that if your blood is high in BPA, your children's blood will likely be high in BPA too.

In response to increasing knowledge surrounding the negative health effects of BPA, many plastic manufacturers have come out with BPA-free options. However, research published in *Current Biology* in 2018 shed light on the fact that these plastics come with their own health problems, like decreased fertility.

Rather than relying on BPA-free plastics, the best course of action is to swap out as much plastic for glass or stainless steel as possible. Ditch plastic food storage containers, plastic bags, plastic wraps, and plastic water bottles. As an added bonus, you'll be helping the environment along with your gut.

#184

GET OUT OF THAT CHAIR

In 2019, statistics showed that the average American adult sits for six and a half hours per day. Since then, there's been a rise in remote work (and longer workdays) that likely have adults sitting for far longer than that. Aside from the fact that sitting too much has been connected to an increased risk of heart disease, stroke, diabetes, high blood pressure, high cholesterol, and dementia, too much time spent in your office chair can also negatively affect your gut health.

Sitting for long periods compresses the muscles in your abdomen, slowing down digestion and leading to digestive issues like bloating, heartburn, and constipation. But when you stand, your abdomen is stretched out, and your bowel functions more efficiently. Researchers from a 2003 study published in *Gut* also found that gas moves through the intestines more quickly when you're standing versus when you're in a seated or lying position, which can improve bloating and flatulence.

As an added bonus, standing while you work has been shown to increase productivity, concentration, and focus, which means you may be able to get more done in a shorter amount of time—a win-win. If you can't switch to a standing desk, make it a point to get up and stretch as often as possible. Set the timer on your phone to go off every thirty minutes. When it does, get up and stretch for a minute or two before getting back to work.

SCALE BACK ON EXERCISE INTENSITY

When it comes to exercise, harder and faster isn't always better, especially if you have gut issues. Exercise is a stressor, and even though it's classified as good stress, sometimes things take a turn for the worse.

Highly strenuous exercise has been shown to:

- Contribute to intestinal permeability, or leaky gut
- Increase cortisol levels (which also contributes to leaky gut)
- Decrease levels of good gut bacteria and promote the growth of bad bacteria
- Reduce blood flow to the gut, which reduces gut motility (movement)

This doesn't mean that you can't ever do intense exercises, but if you're under a lot of stress already or your body doesn't handle stress well, it may be a good idea to scale back for a while or alternate high-intensity days with lower-intensity exercises like yoga, stretching, and/or walking. These lower-intensity exercises reduce inflammation, improve digestion, and get the fluids in your body—like lymph—moving.

What classifies as intense exercise depends on your fitness level, your overall stress load, and how your body responds to stress. As a general rule, intense exercise is defined as anything that raises your heart rate to 70 to 85 percent of its maximum. When you do intense exercises, do them only in short bursts—a minute or two—and make sure you're giving your body enough breaks so that you don't burn out.

#186

HAVE A DAILY ROUTINE

According to a study published in the *Journal of Personality and Social Psychology*, every time you have to make a decision, you increase your stress levels a little bit. The more decisions you have to make, the higher your stress levels get, and the less self-control you have. And just as it negatively affects the rest of your body, stress wreaks havoc on your gut.

But you can take your stress levels down a notch by creating a routine that you stick to every day. Since you'll already know what you'll be doing each day, this limits the number of decisions you have to make and frees up your mental power for other things.

Here are some tips for creating a daily routine:

- Decide what time you'll wake up and stick to that every day, even on the weekends.
- Start your day with something that helps calm your nervous system, like a few minutes of reading or meditating. Try to avoid using your phone, scrolling through social media, or watching the news.
- Remove excess choice as much as possible. Get your clothes ready for the day the night before, plan your meals, schedule dinnertime—plan out all these little things to make your life easier.
- Write down your routine so you can easily see it and reference it (and check things off if you want to).

#187

START YOUR DAY WITH SUN

Sunlight has a powerful effect on your physiology. When your brain senses sunlight, it decreases your body's production of melatonin, a hormone that regulates your sleep-wake cycle. It doesn't just have an immediate effect, though. Exposing yourself to sunlight first thing in the morning also improves your sleep later that night.

Good sleep is important to maintaining optimal gut health, but deficiencies in melatonin have also been linked to leaky gut, while elevated levels of melatonin have been shown to help gut bacteria grow and multiply.

Balancing your melatonin levels through exposure to sunlight has also been shown to help improve symptoms of premenstrual syndrome and seasonal affective disorder (SAD), a type of depression that occurs in the winter months when there's less sunlight throughout the day. Exposure to sunlight in the morning also increases serotonin, a neurotransmitter that contributes to better mood and helps optimize gut health. Low levels of serotonin have been linked to irritable bowel syndrome as well as depression.

Rather than just opening up your curtains, go outside for a few minutes and feel the sun on your face or your bare skin, if you can. Your body is most sensitive to sunlight within the first hour of waking up, so get outside within this time frame for the greatest effect. This effect is even more powerful when you expose yourself to sunlight at the same time each morning, so try to make it a regular, scheduled part of your routine.

DIM THE NIGHT LIGHTS

Just as your brain is most sensitive to the effects of light within the first hour of waking up, it's also very sensitive to light within two hours of going to sleep. Couple this with the fact that many people spend the time right before bed watching TV or scrolling through social media, and it's no wonder that fifty million to seventy million Americans are chronically sleep-deprived (and have a combined total of eighty different sleep disorders).

The best course of action is to avoid any artificial light within two hours of bedtime, but it's unrealistic to think that you'd just sit there in the dark, so here are some other things you can do to help improve your sleep, your hormonal balance, and your gut health:

- Dim the lights in your house or turn off as many as possible.
- Wear blue light–blocking glasses.
- Turn down the brightness on your screens (phones, computers, TVs).
- Install an app on your devices that automatically changes the light "temperature" during certain hours.
- If you have an iPhone, you can turn on "Night Shift" under the Display & Brightness setting or use the manual toggle to change your phone's warmth.
- Use dim red lights for night lights. Red light has less of an effect on melatonin and your circadian rhythm than blue light.

BAN YOUR PHONE FROM THE BEDROOM

If you're like pretty much everyone else in the world, it's highly likely that your phone goes with you wherever you go—to work, to the bathroom, and even to bed.

You know the routine: You swear you're going to bed early tonight, so you take your evening bath or shower, get into some comfy clothes, settle into your bed at 9 p.m., and then scroll through Instagram until midnight. Now you're only going to get six and a half hours of sleep instead of the nine and a half you had planned, and you didn't even realize it was happening. Unfortunately, this mindless scrolling is common, but it can really do a number on your gut health by negatively affecting your sleep.

The simple solution to this would be to not check your phone at night before bed, but that's easier said than done. When your phone is right next to you, it creates a subconscious hypervigilance that makes it hard to ignore notifications. And if you happen to wake up in the middle of the night and can't sleep, even checking the time on your phone exposes you to blue light that interferes with your sleep and can throw off your hormones and circadian rhythm.

Instead, make it a point to keep your phone out of your bedroom at night. If you currently use your phone as your wake-up call, invest in an old-school alarm clock that you can use instead.

#190

WAKE UP SLOWLY

If you have to be up at a certain time in the morning, the current standard is to set an alarm, likely on your phone, that blares a high-pitched sound that startles you awake. Not only does this immediately get your heart racing, it also gets your adrenaline pumping, increases your blood pressure, and sends out a cascade of stress hormones that can throw you, and your gut, off for the entire day. That's no way to start your morning.

Instead, swap out your phone or standard alarm clock for a wake-up light alarm (also called a sunrise alarm clock) that helps you start your day more peacefully. A wake-up light alarm mimics the natural progression of sunlight, waking you up slowly over the course of thirty minutes.

Because light plays a role in your circadian rhythm, this light arousal also sets you up for balanced hormones and a properly functioning digestive system, rather than contributing to stress and gut problems like a blaring noise first thing in the morning.

If you're a heavy sleeper, you may benefit from a wake-up light alarm that comes with a backup sound alarm that you can program to kick in if the light isn't enough to wake you up.

BATHE BEFORE BED

A warm bath (or shower, if you're not into baths) is an excellent way to calm your mind and ease tension in your body and your gut before you head off to bed. The warm water helps relax your muscles—almost instantly, in fact—but there are deeper benefits too.

Warm water activates your body's thermoregulatory system, the physiological system that controls your internal body temperature. About ninety minutes before you go to sleep, your core internal body temperature naturally drops by 0.5°F to 1°F. This temperature drop helps you fall asleep faster and stay asleep longer.

Taking a warm bath or shower to wind down for the night jump-starts that natural thermoregulation process by bringing your body temperature up and then prompting it to dip shortly thereafter, so when it is time to go to bed, you're ready for some serious sleep. And sleeping well helps regulate your circadian rhythm and your stress hormones, which helps keep your gut healthy and happy too.

As little as ten minutes in the bath or shower about an hour or two before bed is enough to do the trick. If you want to really take it up a notch, add some Epsom salt to your bath. The magnesium in the salt helps relax your muscles and your gut, while the warm water gets your body temperature where it needs to be for optimal sleep.

SET THE RIGHT ROOM TEMPERATURE

When it comes to sleeping, everyone has different temperature preferences. Some people like to sleep with the fan on full blast, even in the middle of winter, while others bundle up in flannel pajamas and cover themselves with three layers of blankets. Regardless of your personal preference, experts agree that there's an ideal room temperature for sleeping: 65°F (although anything between 60°F and 67°F should have you snoozing soundly).

This room temperature ensures that your core body temperature won't get too high as you sleep, so you don't toss and turn and get a horrible night of sleep, throwing off your gut in the process.

Here are some tips to make sure your room is the right temperature when it's time for bed:

- Set your thermostat to 65°F.
- Get a quiet fan. A bedroom fan helps circulate air to keep the room cool and feeling fresh.
- Put up blackout curtains. Blackout curtains not only improve sleep by blocking out light, they also block out heat from the sun in the warmer months.
- Wear socks and breathable pj's. Socks help control your body temperature without making you too hot, while fabrics like cotton, linen, and silk allow your body to breathe and don't trap heat as you sleep.
- Avoid exercise too close to bedtime. Not only does exercise raise your body temperature, it speeds up your heart rate and excites your nervous system—all things that make it harder to snooze. Try to work out at least two hours before bedtime.

#193

COOK YOUR OWN MEALS

There's no doubt about it, takeout is tempting, especially after a long day. But even fast foods and convenience foods that are prepared with "healthy" cooking methods can have hidden ingredients that aren't the best choices for your gut health. However, when you cook most of your meals, you can control what goes into your food and make the choices that support your gut rather than contribute to throwing off your microbiome.

You can also control the serving size. Instead of eating the double-sized portion that you get from your favorite restaurant, you can eat a little bit at a time and comfortably fill yourself up without feeling overstuffed and bloated. Cooking at home has also been shown to help improve mood, boost self-esteem, and serve as a powerful stress reliever (assuming you can find a way to enjoy it instead of stress out about it).

You don't have to get fancy—bake some chicken breasts and toss some roasted vegetables in olive oil and you're done—but cooking as many meals as you can at home will naturally help support your gut health, since you tend to use more whole foods when you're cooking from scratch.

Make sure to stick to foods that are as close to their natural form as possible. Limiting processed foods is a major part of supporting your gut health, and making it a point to cook with fresh, whole ingredients as much as possible will do wonders for you.

#194

USE YOUR VENTS

If you have a range hood or a cooking vent, make sure it's on every time you're cooking on the stove. Cooking releases various air pollutants, including carbon monoxide and nitrogen dioxide, into the air. Depending on the pans you use, you may also be releasing some volatile organic compounds, or VOCs (nonstick cookware is notorious for this). When your vent hood is on, it sucks these pollutants up and out of your air so that you don't breathe them in.

The hood also sucks up moisture, lowering humidity that can lead to the growth of bad bacteria and mold. If pathogenic bacteria and mold are allowed to grow in your home, it can create a major—and often hidden—problem. Some molds release mycotoxins, a toxic by-product that triggers an immune response that can cause damage to your intestinal lining, disrupt your gut microbiome, and lead to leaky gut.

This same idea should be applied to your bathroom vent every time you take a shower. While showering doesn't release as many toxins—assuming you're using nontoxic personal care products—the steam from a hot shower creates humidity that allows mold and mildew to thrive. Make it a habit to use all of the vent fans in your house. They're there for a reason.

#195

SWAP OUT YOUR COOKWARE

Nonstick pans may be convenient as far as cooking and cleaning goes, but they're a major source of perfluorooctanoic acid (PFOA) and perfluorooctane sulfonate (PFOS), toxic chemicals that have been shown to disrupt your gut's immune system and increase the risk of digestive problems like ulcerative colitis. PFOS can also change the way your gut metabolizes important compounds like amino acids and short-chain fatty acids, both of which play a role in controlling inflammation and the way your metabolism works.

Exposure to these toxic chemicals negatively affects your gut microbiome, killing good bacteria and allowing bad bacteria to grow in numbers. What's more alarming is that research shows that 96 percent of people in the United States have detectable levels of PFOA in their blood, and even low doses have been shown to have a negative effect.

While you can't completely reduce your exposure to all chemicals, it's important to control what you can. One of the easiest ways to reduce your exposure to PFOA and PFOS is to swap your nonstick cookware for stainless steel, cast iron, or ceramic versions. If you choose a high-quality set, you'll be surprised at how nonstick cookware can be without the toxic coating.

DECORATE WITH PLANTS

Indoor plants not only lift your spirits and decrease stress (two things that improve your gut health over time), but they also have direct physical effects on your gut and your environment. Plants remove volatile compounds, including carbon dioxide and ozone, from your air. And if you remember from elementary school biology, they turn carbon dioxide into oxygen, something that can improve air quality, especially in small spaces that tend to get stuffy.

Plants—and the soil they're grown in—also contain trillions of bacteria (both good and bad), just like your gut. Many of these microbes are similar, meaning they're in your gut *and* on the plant. While many people think it's beneficial to stay away from dirt, exposing yourself to these bugs via your plant's soil helps keep your gut microbiome naturally balanced.

Any plants can have this effect, but the plants with the best purifying qualities include:

- Boston fern
- Spider plant
- Ficus tree
- Bamboo palm
- Lady palm

If you're new to indoor gardening, choose low-maintenance varieties that don't need a lot of light or water. Once you get the hang of taking care of your plants, you can graduate to more advanced plants. Keep in mind that some plants are toxic to animals, so do some research before you head to the nursery if you have pets.

#197

LEAVE YOUR SHOES AT THE DOOR

According to research done by Dr. Charles Gerba, a microbiologist and professor at the University of Arizona, your shoes contain about 421,000 units of bacteria on the outside and 2,887 on the inside. While exposure to different types of bacteria is often a good thing (and your gut contains trillions of units), in this case, the problem is that most of that bacteria is pathogenic and potentially harmful, like *Escherichia coli*, *coliform*, *Klebsiella pneumoniae*, and *Serratia ficaria*—all bacteria that could potentially lead to intestinal and urinary infections. These types of bacteria generally get on your shoes when they come into contact with fecal material, either from public restrooms or animal droppings outdoors. When you wear your shoes in the house, you have the potential to track the bacteria all over your living space.

While the risk that you would actually get sick or develop an intestinal infection from this is pretty low, it's a risk that's not worth taking. If you can support your gut balance and eliminate the risk of pathogenic bacteria getting into your gut just by leaving your shoes at the door, it's a good practice to adopt.

#198

TWEAK YOUR EXERCISE ROUTINE

There's no doubt that exercise is beneficial for your gut, but if you have existing gut issues or uncomfortable digestive symptoms, you may need to tweak your exercise routine. Exercise stimulates digestion, which is a good thing, but if you're in the middle of a HIIT workout or an asana on your yoga mat, you probably don't want to have to poop. These tips can help give you (and your gut) the most comfortable exercise experience possible.

- Avoid eating for about two hours prior to exercise. If you do eat, keep track of your portions. Large meals generally take around two to three hours to digest, while a smaller snack may only need thirty minutes to an hour. Do your workouts after your meals or snacks have finished digesting.
- Limit fatty foods or gas-producing foods, like beans or broccoli, before exercising.
- Avoid caffeine and hot beverages. Both stimulate muscle contractions in the intestines that increase abdominal cramping as you work out.
- Time your workouts for when your intestines are doing the least work, like first thing in the morning or between lunch and dinner.

#199

TURN YOUR WI-FI OFF AT NIGHT

Thanks to the recent introduction of 5G, the world has been buzzing about the potential dangers of electromagnetic fields (EMFs). While you may have written some of this talk off as a conspiracy theory, some research has shown the negative effects that EMFs can have on your gut. While the long-term dangers are still unclear (advanced technology hasn't been around long enough to find out yet), one study published in *Dose-Response* in 2017 found that the EMFs that come from your electronic devices, like your cell phone, laptop, and wireless earbuds, can change your gut microbiome and contribute to the excessive growth of *E. coli*. This can eventually lead to irritable bowel syndrome and/or leaky gut. Another study published in the *Journal of Microbiology* in the same year reported that EMFs negatively affect the balance of bacteria on your skin too.

While it's impossible to completely avoid EMFs nowadays, you can lessen your exposure by turning your Wi-Fi off at night when you're not using it. It's also a good idea to keep your phone as far away from your body as possible and to put it on airplane mode when you're sleeping. If you really want to commit to reducing your exposure to EMFs in your house, you can get rid of Wi-Fi completely and connect to the Internet using an ethernet cable that plugs into your computer and your modem.

#200

KICK THE SMOKING HABIT

If you're a smoker, you probably don't need anyone to tell you that it's a good idea to quit. But while there's a lot of focus on how cigarettes negatively affect heart and lung health, there's less of an emphasis on how it damages your gut, an equally important problem.

According to a review published in the *Archives of Microbiology* in 2018, smoking increases bad bacteria (like *Proteobacteria*, *Bacteroidetes*, *Clostridium*, *Bacteroides*, and *Prevotella*), while also decreasing good bacteria (like *Bifidobacterium*, *Lactococcus*, *Actinobacteria*, and *Firmicutes*). Smoking also decreases bacterial diversity in your gut in a way that's very similar to inflammatory bowel disease and obesity.

Smoking causes inflammation, increases oxidative stress, contributes to leaky gut, and changes the pH of your gut. If you want to have the healthiest gut you can, you need to quit smoking—something that, of course, is easier said than done.

In addition to using nicotine replacement therapy to wean yourself off, research shows that hypnosis is helpful for changing the behavioral patterns that prevent you from kicking the habit. If you've tried everything to quit, it's worth checking out a hypnotist to see if he or she can help.

INDEX

IMPROVE YOUR LIFE—
ONE HACK AT A TIME!

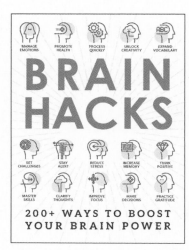

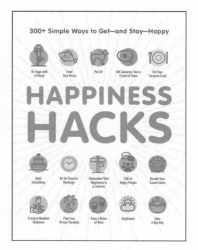

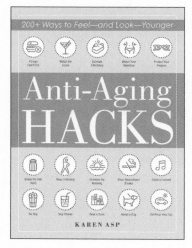

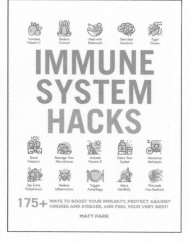

Pick Up or Download Your Copies Today!